Research methods for nurses and the caring professions

Roger Sapsford and Pamela Abbott

Open University Press
Buckingham • Philadelphia

Open University Press
Celtic Court
22 Ballmoor
Buckingham
MK18 1XW

and
1900 Frost Road, Suite 101
Bristol, PA 19007, USA

First Published 1992

A catalogue record of this book is available from the British Library

Library of Congress Cataloging-in-Publication Data

Sapsford, Roger
    Research methods for nurses and the caring professions / by Roger Sapsford and Pamela Abbott.
      p.   cm.
    Includes bibliographical references and index.
    ISBN 0-335-09620-4 (pb)   ISBN 0-335-09621-2 (hb)
    1. Nursing—Research—Methodology. 2. Social service—Research—Methodology. 3. Nursing—Research—Evaluation. 4. Social service—Research—Evaluation.   I. Title
    [DNLM: 1. Nursing Research—methods. 2. Research Design. WY 20.5 S241r]
    RT81.5.S26 1992
    610.73'072—dc20
    DNLM/DLC
    for Library of Congress   91-46382
                                                            CIP

Typeset by Colset (Pte) Ltd
Printed in Great Britain by Biddles Ltd., Guildford and Kings Lynn

Contents

List of exercises

Preface

This is a book on the appreciation and evaluation of other people's research and on the conduct of your own. It stands by itself, but may also be read in conjunction with Pamela Abbott and Roger Sapsford (1992) *Research into Practice: a reader for nurses and the caring professions*, published by Open University Press, which contains many of the examples which are discussed here. One of the book's main aims is to 'de-mystify' research – to distinguish the often complex techniques from the basically fairly simple logic which underlies research projects. The focus is explicitly on *social* research: we shall not be attempting to cover research methods in biology nor research into the efficacy of drugs. The principles are the same, however (except that social research tends to face more complex questions, because of the great variability of its subjects and the fact that the researcher is a part of the social world which he or she is investigating). Most of the examples are small-scale studies, in the sense that they could be (and in many cases were) carried out by one or two people rather than large and well resourced teams. We give particular emphasis to evaluative research of various kinds and the attempt to assess the efficacy of one's own professional practice.

Part of the target audience for this book is the nursing profession – people taking nursing degrees and diplomas, people taking post-qualificatory diplomas and certificates, and practising nurses who want to undertake research or the evaluation of their practice. For this reason a good proportion of the examples are based around the concepts of health and treatment. The book is also appropriate, however, for other community and institutional practitioners, and trainees – for example, social workers, family workers, community workers. The intended level is introductory and you should not imagine that reading it will fully equip you to carry out research of all kinds. There should be enough here to get you started, however, and the rest comes with practice, further reading and competent supervision by others who are already experienced.

The book falls into four sections. The first chapter is a 'mini-course', looking at most of the major ways of collecting data and structuring research and evaluation, and raising many of the issues to which you will come back again and again as you progress through the book. Chapters 2–7 are about reading and evaluating other people's research – Chapter 2 is about the structure of research reports in general, and the others each take a type of research design and examine it through two or three major projects which have used it. Then Chapters 8–14 are on various aspects of the practice of research. The examples range more widely here, but some of them will be taken from the kinds of project that have been carried out by students and could be carried out by you. Finally, there is a chapter on the writing of research reports, and a final summary chapter which also raises and pulls together more fundamental questions about ideology, discourse and the way in which the taken-for-granted aspects of everyday life are also taken for granted in research and evaluation studies.

We have provided practical exercises to back up the text wherever we can. If you are able to fit them into your lives, we strongly recommend trying to carry out the exercises, at the point at which they occur in the text; no amount of descriptive rhetoric is as illuminating as even a small-scale attempt at actually *doing* the research. The exercises are often quite short. Many of them either take no real time at all – they are fitted into time that you would be spending travelling from one place to another, for example – or can be accomplished in 10–20 minutes. Very few of them require any special arrangements or disturbance to your life, except when it is required that you ask someone direct questions, in which case you have to line up someone who is prepared to answer them – often a spouse, or friend or working colleague. (The 'taken-for-granted' in the exercises is that you are able to leave the home in order to go to work or to the shops. If you are entirely housebound then you may need to modify some of them, e.g. observing family interaction rather than the interactions in shops or hospitals, but the exercises so modified will still make the points for which they were designed.) The exercises provided in Chapters 1 and 8–14 are practical activities. In Chapters 3–7 the exercises involve reading and commenting on particular research reports. These may mostly be obtained in academic libraries, or all of them may be found in Abbott and Sapsford (1992), the Reader mentioned above.

Various of the chapters also end with 'Further Reading'. This is not necessary for the understanding of the text, but is intended to expand your horizons beyond what we have written. In Chapters 3–7 the 'Further Reading' suggests other articles or books you might like to examine if the subject area of one of the examples is particularly relevant to your interests or to your area of professional expertise – in other words, to research which you might be interested in carrying out. In Chapters 8–14 we mostly suggest further textbooks or articles, which offer a more detailed treatment than space permits here, of the relevant research techniques, plus a few studies worth reading because they use non-standard and imaginative ways of applying the method. These are not 'required' reading for the chapters, but additional material you will find useful if you go on to do research for yourself in the relevant area and/or style.

Finally, we should acknowledge our colleagues at the Open University, Polytechnic South West and elsewhere, with whom we have been teaching this material and discussing these issues over a long period of years. We are not aware of having 'borrowed' any of their ideas, but all academic work is an unacknowledged collaboration, and we have benefited greatly from having talked and worked with them. We can at least be sure, however, that the mistakes and unorthodoxies are mostly our own.

≡ **Section 1** ≡

Introduction

≡ 1 ≡

Finding out and making sense

'Research' is often presented as something mysterious and technical, something beyond the capability of those who have not undergone long training. It is what is done by scientists, it requires the use of computers and abstruse mathematics, and ordinary untrained people sometimes cannot even understand the questions, let alone the answers. However, 'doing research' is just an extension of what we all do in our daily lives. We are continually coming to conclusions on the basis of what we experience plus what we knew already – to recognize something as a tree, or a postbox or a person is to take knowledge which we have already and apply it to what appears to be in front of us. We all have occasion, every day, to try to find out more about something in order to act more appropriately – to look up an address, to take a closer look at the tree, to explore whether this person is really to be trusted. When something puzzles us and we cannot quite make it out, we generally set about looking for evidence about it which will help us to make sense of it. The researcher does no more. Research starts as an extension of common sense – finding out about things, looking for information about them, trying to make sense of them in the light of evidence and working out what evidence is needed.

Common sense has its limitations, however, which the researcher tries to overcome. In our everyday thinking and decision-making we often act on poor evidence. Indeed, we *have* to do so; events will not wait until the evidence is in, even if we were prepared to collect it. We come to quite hasty judgements about people, for instance, on the basis of one incident; we classify them as sympathetic or unsympathetic on the basis of how they behave when we first meet them, and behave accordingly. We judge whole classes of people on the basis of single examples. Common sense is full of 'facts' for which it has little or no evidence. What has been heard on the radio or television, or in the pub or the bus-queue, or what is believed and announced by opinion leaders such as politicians, churchmen or scientists, becomes 'the truth' without further examination. Finally, common sense is influenced by a wide range of stereotypes and ideological presuppositions of which we are hardly ever aware. Our attitudes to the stranger, to the deviant minority, to those who might be seen as attacking our interests, are so well rooted as to be often impervious to the penetration of logic and evidence. The way we view the world is itself often open to question. Our acceptance of our particular culture's construction of social class, gender and age as supposedly innate or inevitable stratifying principles, together with all the assumptions about people and their wants and needs which these entail, are taken for granted as common sense.

Good research tries not to take for granted what is taken for granted by common sense. It tries to argue rigorously, according to the 'rules of evidence' which we shall be exploring in the rest of this book. At the same time, it requires a degree of imagination, and the power to put the taken-for-granted to one side and 'make the familiar strange'. It is not the *techniques* of research which make it hard work, as you will see in the rest of this book, but the strain of trying to see topic areas simultaneously from all possible angles.

This chapter begins the book with a brief and cursory review of a wide variety of research activities, organized around the ideas of 'looking to see what is going on', 'asking questions' and 'trying something out'. We shall mostly be concerned here with questions of structure in research – structure in the way that questions are asked, or observations or measurements carried out, and structure in the sense of planned comparison between one group and another to illuminate their differences. These are two dimensions along which research studies may differ. (A third major factor – how typicality or representativeness is guaranteed so that you can assert that what is true in the research context is true of the wider population – is left for consideration elsewhere in the book.)

Research is carried out for a wide variety of audiences. Much of what people think of as research – the kind of work carried out by 'researchers' – is to do with the evaluation of new or existing practices. Research is carried out to evaluate the outcome of a policy initiative or the functioning of an existing policy. For example, there will be a fair amount of research published in the next few years on how cash-limited budgets affect the general practice of medicine, and on the functioning of hospitals before and after opting to become 'hospital trusts'. In today's political climate of 'value for money', research is undoubtedly also being carried out into the effectiveness of the health visitor policy of doing home visits to all homes with young children and on whether the expense is justified by what they do there. The effectiveness of treatments is evaluated by controlled research projects: the use of these is most obvious in the clinical trial of new drugs, but similar projects have also been run on the effectiveness of forms of psychological counselling, the introduction of new nursing practices and on innovations in social work practice. 'Before-and-after' projects are also carried out on social innovations (changes in forms of welfare benefits, for example) and gross demographic changes such as the increased life-span of the population (on the 'clients' who are affected by them and the work of the professionals who try to help them).

A second major audience for research is the academic world. Much research is carried out not with the immediate aim of informing policy or practice, but to build an understanding of the field of study and to test theories about it which are derived from more general sociological, psychological or economic models of how the social world is structured and how people function within it. Much of the classic work on health inequalities by region, class and gender, for example, may have been commissioned by government or more local authorities, but has as its aim the discovery of factors associated with poor health and specifically whether the state of health of a group is more affected by their personal actions or by their position within society as defined by structural variables, such as class, gender and material deprivation. (This kind of research blurs into the more 'practical' work discussed in the last paragraph, of course; much social theory is directly concerned with the implementation of social policy.)

A third kind of work involves the evaluation of professional practice. (A fourth kind, less often thought of as 'research', but requiring all the same techniques, is the work of *self*-evaluation.) Research techniques can be used to evaluate the effectiveness of our own practice or that of others, and to test the effects of altering some aspect of it. They can be used to explore the wants and needs of client groups, so that practice can be better informed. They can be used in a vaguer but still rigorous way just 'to find out a bit more about' client groups and working environments, to see if any ideas are generated which may be of use in our practice. This is something we all do without thinking of ourselves as 'carrying out research', but we can do it better if we apply a little rigour and logic. In many ways what distinguishes research from the common-sense use of argument and evidence is a certain 'cast of mind' – an openness to evidence and a distrust of presuppositions, even when taking this critical stance can be personally uncomfortable. When evaluating the work of others – whether their usual way of doing things or some innovative technique – we must clearly be seen to pass judgement fairly, without preconceived ideas, and on the basis of evidence.

In the rest of this chapter we shall be looking at some of the main ways in which evidence is gathered – observation, asking questions, and controlled trials. Practical exercises are provided for you to carry out, and you should endeavour to find time for them if you possibly can; words on paper are no kind of substitute for actually doing some practical work and experiencing both the pleasures of research and its difficulties. If possible, the practical activities should be carried out at the point in the chapter at which they occur, as the experience of them often acts to introduce or reinforce some teaching point which we want to make.

Observation

The most obvious way of getting to know a situation is to go and observe it, and observation is a major way by which research data are collected. Just how to *do* observation, however, is not quite as obvious as it might at first appear. Events are not just 'there' for us to note as if we were cameras taking pictures.

On the contrary, in a sense we construct our world as we observe it, seeing what we do as a result of the knowledge which we already have. The same 'event' could be a parent disciplining a child in one frame of observation, a case of child abuse in another, and a piece of play-acting in a third. It could also be analysed in terms of local norms of parental discipline, patterns of communication or even patterns of physical movement. (One can – just about! – imagine a sports physiotherapist who was more interested in whether the muscles of the arm were working smoothly than in whether the hand was causing pain.) Similarly, there are many different ways of observing in research, good for different purposes and with different drawbacks.

Exercises 1–6: Observation

These exercises will take about 30 minutes, not including time spent taking notes. They do not have to be done all at once; they are split up into 5-minute 'sessions', and each session could be done on a different day if that were more convenient for you.

Find yourself somewhere where the general public gather for some purpose and interact with someone who is in some kind of service or regulatory role. If you work in a hospital or general medical practice or in a social services department you may be able to observe a 'reception area' where people wait around for their appointments. If you are a health visitor you may be able to do your observation in a clinic. Parents may be able to observe other parents at 'mums and toddlers' groups. Otherwise, a good location is a large self-service shop where people take their own goods from shelves and queue at a cash-desk to pay for them. Whatever the location, you want somewhere where you can stand around for 5 minutes at a time without drawing attention to yourself; those under observation must not know that you are observing, and if you are observing in a shop you will not want to be suspected as a potential shop-lifter.

All the sessions require you to take notes. For the first two you will want to go away somewhere to do this – sit outside, or go and have a cup of coffee. The others require you to record numbers of various kinds, so you will need to take notes while actually doing the observation. Work out how to do this unobtrusively beforehand – in a small notebook, perhaps, or on what might be taken for a shopping list, or on a magazine or the margins of a book.

Exercise 1
Spend 5 minutes just looking round and seeing what is going on in general. At the end of the 5 minutes, go and sit down somewhere, and write some notes on what you have seen – not more than a page, but at least eight or ten lines, describing what was going on.

Exercise 2
Spend another 5 minutes focusing on the cashier or receptionist (without attracting his or her attention), looking at how he or she deals with people, how the people behave and whether they appear satisfied, disconcerted or annoyed by the

interchange. Again, go somewhere and write some notes on what you have seen.

Exercise 3
Now spend another 5 minutes (or as long as it takes to get at least 10 interchanges between the cashier/receptionist and a member of the public) looking at what is done in each interchange. Count how many of the interchanges involve one or both parties speaking, whether the cashier/receptionist appears to treat them in a friendly, distant or haughty manner, and whether the members of the public appear polite, rude, brusque or neutral with respect to him/her.

Exercise 4
For another 5 minutes (or 10 interchanges), count the total amount of time spent speaking in the interchanges by (a) the cashier/receptionist, (b) male members of the public and (c) female members of the public. Count slowly to yourself at a constant speed while any speech is occurring and jot down the numbers in three columns, to be totalled later.

Exercise 5
Spend 5 minutes concentrating on the cashier/receptionist, and count the number of seconds he or she spends looking at the face of the member of the public with whom he or she is interacting.

Exercise 6
Finally, go to another kind of location and repeat the count you have just done on a different cashier/receptionist. If you used a waiting room of some kind for your main location, go to a shop for this last part of the exercise. If you used a shop, try observing in a library or a garage or at the ticket-office of a large railway station.

The notes from the first exercise, where you were recording simply 'what was going on', would probably tell us more about you than about the events which you were observing. What we asked you to do, effectively, was to make sense of the situation, and you will have done so largely in terms of your own well-tried and pre-existing categories. It is possible that what actually happened may have surprised you, but nonetheless you will have described the situation in terms which came readily to you and made sense to you. You can see, however, that this kind of 'holistic' observation – trying to make sense of situations as a whole – is not as easy as it looks, and that more careful work needs to be done before the conclusions are readily acceptable as evidence. When we come to look at this kind of observation later in the book, you will see that it generally involves quite long periods of immersion in a situation, as a person with a role within it rather than just as a 'neutral' observer.

The second exercise may have taxed you more, because we asked you to concentrate on one participant for five minutes, a longer span of attention by far than you would normally grant to one person with whom you were not in interaction. This being so, we suspect you probably came to regard what was going on as to some extent strange – to start describing it to yourself in different terms from the ones that you would use in everyday life – and to that extent you may have come up with something which surprised you and would surprise us. Making the familiar strange is one stance regularly adopted by researchers who wish to penetrate below the taken-for-granted aspects of the situation. However, note that the closer focus on the cashier/receptionist in itself imposes structure on what you may have 'seen'; you were asked to focus on an individual, so you undoubtedly came up with notes bearing on the actions of that individual and the actions taken towards him or her, and with very little on the more general and structural features of the situation.

Exercises 3–6 introduced a new dimension by asking you to *count* something. What you counted became increasingly more specialized. What the numbers allow you to do is to provide a more convincing and 'available' description of the situation. We no longer have to depend on your judgement as to what was going on, however good and reliable that might be; you present us with figures on some aspect of the situation, and we can look at them for ourselves. In Exercise 4, for example, we can see whether men spoke more than women, not just accept your judgement that one or the other gender was more active, and compare the activity of clients with the activity of the 'gate-keeper'. Comparing Exercises 5 and 6, we can look at the different behaviour of 'professionals' in two contrasting situations, as judged from an aspect of behaviour which has been shown to be very important in the regulation of face-to-face relationships.

Looking back over what you have collected, you will probably find that the data from the later exercises were much more 'definite' than what was collected in the earlier ones. ('Data' means 'what has been collected for analysis' – in the early exercises your notes on what happened, and in the later exercises the counts that you made.) Figures seem somehow to carry more weight in an argument than one's vaguer general impressions, to look more like 'proof', to seem somehow more 'neutral' than more general descriptions. You will realize already, however, that there is nothing magic about numbers as such. Numbers can, indeed, be more precise, and it is certainly easy to argue from them that something is more common than something else, or that two somethings are related. The value of the numbers, however, is created at the stage of data-collection, and it depends entirely on your accuracy (how good were you at counting seconds?) and on what we decided to count in the first place. If what we decided to count was not important, then the data will be of no importance, irrespective of how neatly laid out in numbers they are. We constructed the situation as one in which speech and eye-contact were 'the important thing that was going on'. All manner of interesting actions may have taken place during the interactions, but in the later exercises you will not know what they were. (At least, *you* may know what went on, but they do not appear in your data and are, therefore, not available for subsequent analysis.) Different frames of analysis – in terms of economic exchange, multi-person systems, personal histories, structural inequalities, etc. – are effectively ruled out by the way in which we elected to collect the data in the earlier exercises.

Thus, there are many forms of observation, ranging from the very general and unstructured to the very structured and numerical. None of them is necessarily the 'right' way to proceed; each has advantages and disadvantages for particular situations, depending on your aims as a researcher and what you know already. We shall explore observation techniques in more detail in later chapters.

Asking questions

Another obvious and everyday way of proceeding, if you want to know what is going on and what people are thinking, is to ask them. A great deal of social science research is concerned with the asking of questions, and a substantial technology, folklore and body of expertise has grown up around the art and science of asking them. We ask a lot of questions as part of our everyday conversations. Ordinary everyday conversation can be a prime source of information and you might well be taking advantage of it as part of a relatively unstructured piece of observation research. If you were studying a hospital ward without the people there knowing you were doing research – pretending to have an official role there, for example, or actually being a nurse and observing your own workplace – then part of the data you would collect would be what people said to you. If you were participating but being open about the fact that you were a researcher you could ask more questions, and more obvious ones; indeed, you would be expected to do so by the other participants. The strength of this kind of ordinary, everyday questioning is that you get what the participants want to say, in their own words and using their own concepts.

The problem with ordinary conversation is that you contribute as much to it as does the person to whom you are talking. Indeed, as it is you who are asking the questions, you will probably contribute *more* of the ideas that matter; it will be you that 'starts the ball rolling' with each topic, and the terms in which you do so are likely to structure the subsequent exchanges. So, far from getting the participant's own ideas in his or her words, you will get your own words and ideas fed back to you. An example which springs to mind is a student whom one of us was supervising on a methods course who was asking questions about social class and how the informant saw the social world as being structured. The informant used a categorization of working-class people into 'rough' and 'respectable', which the student found quite exciting, because it duplicated a set of categories which have been in use for over a hundred years and underlies the practice of charitable and state welfare – the distinction between the deserving and the undeserving poor. Checking back over the transcript of the interview, however, he found that he had been the first person to introduce this distinction, without thinking or noticing. The informant had found it a useful one and had used it consistently thereafter. So the student had no notion of how the informant would have described the world if this set of categories had not been made available.

When we 'interview' people rather than just chatting to them, we tend to play down our own part in the interview, to say as little as possible, to put across as few ideas new to the informant as possible and to concentrate on eliciting the pre-existent ideas of the informant in the informant's own words. This kind of interviewing is a very common means of research into social topics. It is often used to contrast groups of people who differ in some key respect or to compare the same people over time, and before and after major policy changes or 'social landmarks'. You will find it referred to in the literature as 'ethnographic', 'qualitative', 'semi-structured' or 'unstructured' interviewing. We did not like any of these terms, so we have coined the term 'open interviewing' to describe it.

So much for 'open' interviewing. There is also a more systematic and structured way of asking questions – you will probably be most familiar with it from being stopped by market-research interviewers in the street – which uses predesigned questionnaires or schedules. (A *questionnaire* is a list of questions for self-completion by the respondent; an *interview schedule* is a list of questions to be asked by an interviewer, face to face or on the telephone.) These are used in national surveys such as the Census for obtaining factual information from respondents – number of people in household, number of rooms in the house, etc. Their purpose is to collect exactly comparable information from every respondent, on a large scale. It is obviously important in the Census, for example, that the interviewers and respondents have a precise definition of what constitutes a household, and the same definition for every respondent. Otherwise, if the same group of people sharing a flat might be classified as one household in one part of the country and a number of co-resident single households in another, then we would be collecting information not about patterns of domestic living, but about whether people *think* of themselves as a household or not. Even an apparently simple question such as the number of rooms in house needs very precise definition. Does the bathroom count as a room? What about a separate and very small w.c., or a shower cubicle *en suite* to a bedroom? Is a breakfast room with a kitchen alcove to count as one room or two?

Structured questionnaires and interview schedules are also used for the collection of information about attitudes, beliefs and intentions. The kind with which you are likely to be most familiar are market-research interviews – 'What do you think of this product?' – and political opinion polls – 'Which political party would you vote for if there were a General Election today?' Similar kinds of questionnaires are also used extensively by social psychologists and sociologists to test theories about the relationship of attitudes to each other, and they are one standard way of assessing likely popular reaction to policy changes. Their merit is that a great deal of data can be collected relatively quickly, and that the same questions are asked of everyone, allowing comparisons to be drawn. It is also possible, under certain conditions, to generalize with some degree of precision from a sample to the population as a whole; this is discussed in Chapters 6 and 9. There are corresponding disadvantages, however, as the following exercises may help to make clear.

Exercises 7 and 8: Interviewing

Exercise 7
Find some-one who is prepared to sit down with you in a quiet place for a quarter of an hour or so – a friend or spouse will do – and ask him or her the following list of questions:

(For questions a–c, do not offer definitions or explanations. If asked, say 'Whatever you yourself mean by "healthy" ' etc.)

(a)	Would you regard yourself as a healthy person?	Yes No	(Ring one)
(b)	Are you often ill?	Yes Seldom No	(Ring one)
(c)	Have your ever suffered from a serious disease?	Yes Seldom No	(Ring one)

(For question d show the respondent the scale – perhaps copied out on a piece of paper. Do not explain or offer definitions: say 'Whatever you yourself mean by . . .'.)

(d) Could you please indicate the state of your health on a scale from 1 to 7?

1	2	3	4	5	6	7
Very healthy	Fairly healthy	Mostly healthy	Neither healthy nor unhealthy	Occasionally unhealthy	Often unhealthy	Mostly unhealthy

(e) How old are you? --- (Write in)

(For question f, say 'for any reason whatsoever' if asked to clarify.)

(f) How often have you been to the doctor in the last year? _____ times (Write in)

(For question g, check that time spent waiting because the respondent arrived early is not counted.)

(g) How long did you have to wait before getting in to see him or her, on the last occasion?

1	2	3	4	5	6	9
Not at all	Up to 5 mins	5–15 mins	16–30 mins	31–60 mins	More than an hour	Can't remember

(h) What was the purpose of your visit? -------------------------- (Write in)

Exercise 8
Now talk to your respondent for 5 or 10 minutes – or rather, get him or her to talk to you – about the trip to the doctors and his or her health in general. Encourage the informant to speak freely.

The interview schedule you used in Exercise 7 is obviously a very short one, made up for the occasion, but it does display the major forms of question used. Questions a–c are essentially yes/no questions, though b and c offer a mid-point. (Did you have difficulty trying to get the respondent to say 'yes' or 'no' to question a?) Question d is an attitude scale. Questions e and f ask for a straightforward number. Question g again asks for a number, but the answer is recorded as a *code*, a number standing in for a range of possible answers. In question h you just write down (in summary form) whatever reason the respondent gives; this would be coded afterwards into categories.

The importance of clear instruction to ensure comparable responses is also evident. In most of the questions you were instructed not to offer definitions or explanations, but to force the respondent to make up his or her own mind what the questions meant. This would mean that the answers would have to be interpreted in terms of whether respondents think themselves healthy, not against some absolute standard of health. (We could have obtained further information which would have helped the interpretation of the data, however, by asking whether they had suffered from any of a list of diseases and ailments during the last year. Most people would describe themselves as healthy even if they have had a cold, for example, but only some would describe themselves as healthy, but suffering from arthritis.) We were careful to exclude 'unnecessary waiting time' in question g – time spent waiting because the respondent was early for an appointment. There are still ambiguities left in, however; for example, what about home visits from doctors, or times when the respondent visited the surgery, but saw the practice nurse, or visited only to deliver a specimen. At least one of the apparently simple counts is, in fact, fraught with potential error, because it asks for 'number of times in the last year'; people's memories are very unreliable for time-periods such as this. (It might have been better to anchor the time-period to a memorable event – 'how often since Christmas?', for example.) In that same question, you may have had difficulty coding the answer. What did you do, for example, with respondents who initially said 'not very long', or 'absolutely ages', or '15 to 20 minutes'? We didn't give you instructions on whether to probe or not – to ask follow-up questions. Did these responses go down as 'can't remember', or did you probe further to get a figure out of them? What confidence do you have in the figure, if they were vague initially? And note that if several interviewers were all using this schedule on different respondents, and they used different probes, then the answers to this question would not strictly be comparable. Designing structured questionnaires and schedules is not as easy as it may look at first sight.

When you talked with the informant afterwards, in Exercise 8, did you get the feeling that the definition of 'health' and 'healthy' was not the simple, cut-and-dried matter that the interview schedule seems to suggest. Did you, in fact, spend a certain amount of time *negotiating* with the informant what together you were prepared to count as 'being healthy', 'being unhealthy', 'being ill'. Did you find yourself swapping experiences with your informant and describing your own views on health? As you can see, the structured interview data are not nearly as rich and full as what can be collected by open interviewing, nor do they give one complete confidence that the respondent's complex views and life-circumstances are fully recorded. On the other hand, it would not be possible to use open interviewing on a very large sample: it takes too long. Also, you will have seen for yourself just how very difficult it is not to suggest to the informant what you are prepared to count as an acceptable answer – which would mean you were to some extent collecting your own views, not theirs.

Controlled trials

We have repeatedly talked about measurement before and after a change, and this is the key to the more systematic research design known as the 'controlled trial' or 'experiment'. If we want to try out a drug which is expected to reduce pulse-rate, for example, it would not be much evidence of its effectiveness just to give people the drug and then measure their pulse-rate; we could accidentally have picked people whose normal pulse-rate was abnormally low or high. The minimum which would count as reasonable evidence of effectiveness, therefore, is measurements before administering the drug and afterwards, so that we could document a decrease. This is the essence of the experimental approach: a pretest, a treatment or manipulation, and a posttest. Everything else that is built into experimental design represents the experimenter's attempts to show that the change is actually produced by what he or she says it is produced by – that there is no other plausible explanation for it.

In the simple drug experiment which we have just described, the evidence for a change is good, but the evidence that it is the drug which produced it is not very good. Almost anything might be responsible for it; for example, the group could have been taking exercise just before the administration of the drug, in which case we would have expected their pulse to decline from an initial high reading whether or not they took the drug. This kind of obvious physical feature can be controlled for – we simply make sure that it does not occur – but it is impossible to guard against *every* confounding factor, including those which have not even occurred to us. Normal practice, therefore, is to select a second group who go through exactly the same procedures as the first, but do not receive the drug. If pulse declines in the experimental group (the one that received the drug) and not in the control group (the one that did not), then we are on fairly firm ground in arguing that it is the drug that produced the effect.

However, this argument holds only to the extent that the two groups are exactly similar and undergo exactly the same procedures except for the experimental treatment. The experimenter goes to great length to ensure this similarity. Similarity of people is ensured by: 'matching' cases (selecting pairs of people who are the same in key respects) and allocating one from each pair randomly to an experimental or control group; or by jumbling up the names of all the selected subjects, and drawing out an experimental and a control group at random; or sometimes by using the same subjects as control and experimental group. The merits of the three different approaches are discussed in Chapter 10. Similarity of treatment is guaranteed by careful duplication of procedures and by using a little imagination as to what might go wrong.

We have used a drug trial as an example of an experiment because such trials are easy to describe and understand. Precisely the same principles are applied in social experiments, however. Experimental social psychologists run just the same kind of procedure, with experimental and control groups measured beforehand on the variable which the experimenter intends to change, a 'treatment' applied to the experimental group but not the control group, and a post-test to assess the extent of the change produced in one group and not the other. You might use a similar procedure to assess the effects of an innovative nursing or social-work practice or the efficiency of a new teaching method. In the 'scientific' style of experiment, a key question is the accurate measurement of 'variables' – producing numbers which mean something, for subsequent analysis. The same design logic, however, would underlie an evaluation study carried out by one of the more holistic and less measurement-obsessed methods, such as unstructured observation or open interviewing. You would still want to assess how things were before the onset of whatever it was whose effects you were evaluating, and then again afterwards, and you might well include among the people you observed or interviewed a group who were not exposed to the change, to make changes amongst those who did experience it more interpretable by comparison.

Indeed, the same logic underlies many research reports which are not experimental. A frequent form of research involves looking at something which has occurred in one region – a new way of doing health visiting, say – and comparing some supposed outcome of it with how things were in the same region before the change and with how things were at the same points of time in a region where the change has not occurred. This cannot class as an experiment because there is no guarantee that the two groups which are being compared are like each other; regions may differ in the sort of people who live in them. You do have pretests and post-tests in both regions, however, and a 'treatment' administered in one region and not the other. The same form of argument would be used in interpreting the results, therefore, except that more care and investigation would have to go into demonstrating that it was fair to compare the two regions. (We sometimes call this kind of research *quasi*-experimental: it is *like* the experiment and shares its logic, but lacks some of its more important strengths.)

Exercise 9: Field experiment

At some time when you are likely to pass a fair number of people – on your way to work in the morning, for example – try controlling your own behaviour systematically and see if it has any effect on the behaviour of those whom you pass. With the first five people whom you pass, smile at them and look them in the eye. Note whether they smile back or greet you, and jot down the number unobtrusively – perhaps on the margin of a newspaper. (If you pass a group of people, focus on only one of them and do not count the others.) Now, with the next five, do not smile, and look at their chins instead of their eyes. Again, count how many smile at or greet you. Carry on doing this, smiling at five and not smiling at the next five, until you have at least 20 of each. Compare the number who smiled or greeted you in the 'smiling' condition with the number who did so in the 'not smiling' condition.

'Not smiling' is the control condition and 'smiling' the experimental treatment, in this exercise. As it was the same person who did both, we have no problems about comparing them in that respect. However, your journey to work is not uniform in terms of whether you are likely to meet people who already know you. Typically, people start off walking down a street where most people are known to them at least by sight, then get into territory less well frequented by acquaintances, then begin to recognize people again as they get near to where they work. This is why we asked you to do five 'smiles' and five 'no smiles', alternating: that way there is less likelihood that all of the people you pass in the 'smiling' condition would be known to you and all of the others unknown, or *vice versa*. Although only a small exercise, with a trivial 'manipulation', this design in fact shows many key features of the traditional field experiment of social psychology (i.e. one carried out 'in the real world', not in a laboratory or other artificial setting). It might have been set up to test a theory about the control of one person's behaviour by rewarding features of the others. On the other hand, it might have tested what happens when you initiate or do not initiate socially constructed 'greeting sequences' by catching someone's eye and smiling. Note that even where an experiment is technically well constructed, the interpretation of its results may not be unambiguous; in this case, the 'treatment' could be interpreted as two different things – administering a reward or initiating a 'social script' – depending on the theory from which you approach it.

You may also want to think whether the experiment was quite ethical. No particular harm was done to anyone, but it must have been disconcerting to some people to be, in a sense, greeted warmly by a complete stranger who then passed on down the street without following through into conversation. A charge often rightly levelled against those who carry out experimental research is that they are callous or unimaginative about the harm which their procedures might do to their subjects.

On the other hand, the overall *logic* of experimental design underlies all serious attempts to evaluate policy or practice. As we argued above, the logic of experimentation is not particularly tied to one method of data-collection; it can be applied as readily to unstructured observation or open interviewing as to the more structured methods traditionally associated with it. Indeed, it also underlies a fair amount of conventional practice in the caring professions. The Nursing Process, or the Health Visiting Process, are modelled on evaluation studies and draw on their logic. They consist in a pretest (assessment of a 'case' and his or her needs), a decision as to what is to be done, its implementation, and re-assessment to determine the outcome. All that is lacking is a control group or condition. Social-work practice and teaching follow similar lines though in less explicit form; their practice consists in assessment of a situation, action in accordance with the assessment, and re-assessment to evaluate the effects of action.

The research imagination

We have tended to talk on occasions, as everyone does, as if 'research' were a set of skills to be brought out and applied to the particular problem. This is true, of course, but a training in research entails more than this. As we suggested earlier, the 'research stance' is more a frame of mind, an openness and neutrality at the point of immediate argument, a kind of imagination. Few research projects are definitive in the answers they offer, and the unit of research is generally not the particular project – the controlled trial, the interview study, the period of observation – but the whole programme of related studies which explore and expand the question. Our notional drug trial, for example, would not be possible until the drug had been developed as a result of a large series of experimental studies in the pharmaceutical laboratory. Nor would one study be enough to show that it worked and had no harmful side-effects. The good research team would replicate – run the study again, to check that the results did not come up positive by chance alone. They would try the drug out on a wide range of people, to make sure it was safe for all and not just some of them. They would think about possible side-effects and run specific studies to try to detect them in a harmless form before they occurred in clinical practice with potentially fatal consequences. They would follow up all the people who had received the drug, over time, and look for longer-term effects. One question suggests another.

One aspect of the research imagination – particularly important in the more structured and 'quantified' styles of research – is having the imagination to know what data to collect. Open studies (participant observation, open interviewing) can often 'change their own agenda' by bringing up ideas as important which had not occurred to the researcher. More structured studies (questionnaire surveys, structured observation, controlled trials) collect the data which they *do* collect and are not open to surprises. To take an obvious example: if the classic epidemiological research on cancer had not collected information on whether people smoked, it *could not* have shown an association between smoking and lung cancer.

Studies may also lead to the research question being modified and expanded. In the case of the small field experiment you ran on the effect of smiling on the way to work, for example, we came up with two possible explanations – the 'reward characteristics' of smiling, and its function as the beginning of a well-learned social script. If we were developing theory in this area we would want to run at least one further study to determine which of these, if either, was the more useful explanatory concept. In the process we might throw up further possible competing explanations which would need to be explored. We would also be developing our theory of the functions of smiling at the same time, and the developed theory might well suggest further questions which necessitated research. Where the questioning stops is an arbitrary decision; if the theory has merit, it is probably capable of indefinite expansion and refinement.

The researcher who does commissioned research also learns to widen the frame of reference when considering questions of research design. If you had been commissioned by management to study how cashiers in a large shop could improve the impression they gave to customers, or health receptionists the impression they gave to clients, you might well have carried out some or all of the observation studies which we tried out as Exercises 1–6. Management would have framed the question in terms of what cashiers/receptionists do and how they behave, and social psychology's past research on the functions of eye-contact and speech-sharing as satisfying aspects of interaction might well have led you to the kind of studies we proposed in the exercises. The underlying question, however, is not the narrow 'What can cashiers/ receptionists do?', but the broader 'How can things be improved for customers/ clients?', and you might well direct your research to this wider question rather than the narrower way in which management had framed it. The receptionist/ cashier and her behaviour is only one element in the situation. You would have looked at her physical circumstances and whether they were conducive to friendly behaviour. You would have looked at the number of interchanges she had to manage – her work-load – to see whether it was excessive. You would have looked at her rates of pay, and the rates of pay of comparable jobs, and the possibilities for promotion. You might even have regarded long queues as inevitable and looked at what was offered to clients/customers while they were waiting, to 'serve them up' as friendly people at the point of interaction. You would almost certainly have talked to everyone material to the interaction – the cashier/receptionist, the customers/clients, other 'professionals' involved in the scene – to get their views and explore their satisfactions and dissatisfactions.

The broader the frame of reference, within the practical constraints of what can be managed within the available time, the broader the understanding, and broader understanding leads mostly to better solutions. It takes a measure of imagination to conceptualize a problem widely enough to make it really worth doing research on it. It is now some time since the medical profession realized – occasionally – that more needs to be taken into account in drug research than just the biochemical action of the drug. (A famous series of experiments demonstrated that some doctors get better results than others with the same drug, and that some doctors get better results with placebos – inactive pills – than others get with the active drug.) It is now commonplace in the teaching of nurses and health visitors to stress that medical 'facts' about patients exist as just one part of complex social lives and networks of understanding, and that what may seem a good pattern of care from the medical point of view may not be the best form of approach if the 'total patient' is taken into account.

Nonetheless, we lapse into simple thinking – not least in the sphere of medicine and nursing – and run simple studies based on preconceived ideas of what 'must' be the right course of action.

The rest of this book is devoted to studying a range of good research which has already been carried out and to looking for ways in which 'good practice' in research can be applied to the kinds of situations that you might find yourself wanting to explore. We hope that you will bring your widest imagination to the reading and not let anything be 'taken for granted'.

≡ Section 2 ≡

Assessing research

Reading research reports

In this section of the book we shall be considering a range of different kinds of research through reading and analysing a number of published research reports. The current chapter stands as an introduction to this work and looks at the structure of research reports and how best to go about reading them. Some of what we say may on first reading seem abstract and difficult. However, the research skills which we are trying to get across will become clear as you carry on with the rest of the section, read our evaluations of the papers and start to evaluate research reports for yourself.

When we look at particular research reports in Chapters 3–7, a starting point will be a check-list of the topics which we shall discuss briefly in this chapter and consider in more detail in the remainder of the book.

1 Does the design of the research lend itself to the arguments which are based on it – can the conclusions drawn follow logically from what has been done?
2 Could there be other explanations of the results – alternative theorizations which might characterize what has been found in quite different ways?
3 Could the results be due to variables which are 'confounded' in the design – accidentally confused with what we really want to measure? Or could they be an artefact of the research situation?
4 What is measured? Are the measuring instruments valid and reliable? Does the choice of 'quantities' to measure close off certain kinds of explanations and predispose us from the start to other kinds? (This is a series of questions, but they are all closely inter-related.)
5 To what population may the results be generalized?
6 Was anyone harmed, embarrassed or even inconvenienced by the research?
7 To what extent are people treated as objects by the research?
8 In whose interests is the research carried out?

9 Does the way in which the research is framed embody ideological pre-suppositions such that the outcome is 'written in' or 'predetermined' by the original conceptual analysis and design?

10 Are the results of any conceivable interest? Can I use them in my practice?

This is a check-list of the questions that can be asked of research reports. Not all of them are relevant to all reports. You need to ask the questions relevant to the particular paper, which is what we try to do when we evaluate reports in this section of the book. What we have tended to do in discussing each paper is to concentrate on the questions that are most relevant for evaluating that type of research, not every question that could conceivably be raised. (It is also important to bear in mind that the questions we ask of a research report are, in part, determined by the purpose for which we are reading it.)

The structure of reports

A formal research paper is expected to have a simple and readily comprehensible structure. Every paper outlines, in order: what the question or field of investigation is (and, probably, why it is interesting and/or what is already known about it); how the researcher or research team have gone about looking at it; what the results are; and what the results mean. Thus, you can reasonably expect that a published paper aimed at an academic/research/professional audience will consist of:

1 an *Introduction* which sets up the question or problem, explains why it is of interest to theory, policy and/or practice, and probably reviews the 'literature' (previous published reports, etc.) relevant to it;

2 a *Methods* section: how the problem or area is to be explored;

3 a *Results* section: what was found out;

4 a *Discussion* section: what the results mean, what they imply, and any major reasons for treating them with caution.

Books vary more in their precise organization, but you would expect a similar ordering of contents (except that some of the Methods material is often relegated to an Appendix at the end of the work, to save 'ruining the narrative flow').

The form of this kind of report will be familiar to you from school science: it is the format of the school laboratory report ('Method: A pipette was taken . . .'). Not all 'social science' research would think of itself as 'scientific' in this way, but the form of the scientific report is, nonetheless, a good one for presenting research results and showing what may be concluded from them, and it is widely used. This kind of report fits in most naturally with 'quantitative' research – experiments, controlled trials, surveys, systematic observation – but a similar *logic* is followed by reports of research in more 'qualitative' or 'appreciative' styles – open interviews, unstructured participant observation. What these latter tend to add is a greater narrative element, telling the story of the research process in more realistic detail.

Those who adopt a more 'qualitative' research design tend to be more aware of their data as the outcome of a process in which they themselves participated and in which their own attempts to make sense of the situation and those of the other participants will necessarily have had a great effect on what is produced. Thus, qualitative reports tend to display greater *reflexivity*: they reflect more on the process of the research, on how the participants made sense of it, on their own preconceptions, and on how detailed events may have shaped the nature of the data. In fact, you will now find an increasingly reflexive stance taken even in the more scientific style of report, as the proliferation of formal methods courses makes a generation of academics more aware of the extent to which how people make sense of their situation can shape the nature of the data collected. Reflexivity is a quite essential component of the more qualitative research report, however; it is the major means by which we can assure ourselves of the quality of the evidence, given that we were not there when it was collected.

The majority of reports and accounts of research, of course, are not 'research reports'. Most are written for administrators who need to use the results, or for commercial companies, or presented to a relevant audience in a more 'popular' professional publication (e.g. *Nursing Times*, *Social Work Today*, *The Health Visitor*), or reported in the popular press or on radio or television for everyone's consumption. Many of the reports you come across in these ways will not cover all the sections that we outlined above. In particular, 'popular' reports tend to give little or no detail of how the evidence was collected; this is seen as tedious for the lay audience and, therefore, to be avoided. To the extent that such detail is not there, however, we should be very chary of accepting the conclusions which are claimed for the research as anything more than someone's claims. Popular reports tend to expect you to accept conclusions on the authority of the researcher; you are not given the resources to form your own conclusion about their validity.

Assessing reports

In reading a research report and assessing the worth of its conclusions, your first steps will be:

1 to look at the Introduction, to see what the researchers were looking for and why it is supposed to be interesting;
2 secondly, you will look at the Discussion/Conclusions (and perhaps the end of the Results section) to see what the authors claim to have found and what they think it means;
3 with this established we can go on to look a little under the surface of the results and assess the quality of the evidence as well as the quality of the arguments based on it.

Looking at the arguments and the evidence, the first step is clearly to assess their overall validity: do the conclusions follow validly from the initial arguments, given the evidence that is presented? At the same time you need to look at the research part of the paper – the Methods and Results sections – and see if *they* constitute a valid argument. The paper will be arguing that certain kinds of results will be obtained or *not* be obtained, if an initial line of theory is to remain plausible. Or it will be claiming that an account of what a given social setting is like, based on survey methods or on open interviewing or on participant observation, is to be accepted as a valid characterisation of what it is actually like. In either case there is an implicit argument in the project: 'given what I have measured or recorded, the best interpretation of it is the one which I am advancing'. You will be examining this claim very carefully to see whether alternative explanations could be put forward – alternative theories, or explanations based on inadequacies in the design of the research. Questions of reflexivity arise here: is the researcher well enough aware of the likely effect of the procedures on the data, and has he or she given us enough information to judge this? A part of the examination will also cover the question of measurement: are the measuring instruments or methods of recording and classifying observations *valid* – do they measure what the authors claim they measure – and are they *reliable* – are they likely to produce consistent results rather than values which are much at the mercy of chance? These are some of the questions that we shall be exploring with you in the next five chapters, where we look in detail at a relatively small number of concrete research studies.

Another question which will arise in reading some papers – particularly the more 'scientific' ones – revolves around the question of operationalization. Many of the phenomena which the social scientist wants to measure are not readily and obviously available for measurement. What we actually have to measure is something which acts as a 'symptom' of the underlying characteristic – ability to answer questions on paper as an indicator of intelligence, job and/or attitudes (verbal expressions) as indicators of social class, what patients say and what they do as indicators of depression. From these we deduce a measurement for the underlying characteristic. The problem of validity which we mentioned in the last paragraph obviously applies: in translating the theoretical characteristic into something operational that can be measured, do we succeed in producing something which really does measure it? A further problem arises, however. Psychologists take the concept of intelligence for granted, for example, as we all tend now to do, but the idea that people can be placed on a continuum of general ability in this way is quite a recent invention (see Rose 1985), and one which embodies as 'fact' a range of politically very contentious ideas and practices (see Kamin 1974). Sociologists take their ability to place people in social classes for granted, and measures of social class are a commonplace in very down-to-earth projects such as the analysis by market researchers of what newspapers different people read. The way the concept is used, however, often presents as facts some very contentious statements about social inequalities (see Abbott and Sapsford 1987a, for example, for a discussion of the problems and consequences of assigning social class in different ways to married women). So part of the assessment of a piece of research may involve critical analysis of its basic concepts – the apparently unproblematic 'things' which it sets out to measure – to see whether ideological propositions are being put forward unwittingly as unproblematic 'facts', biasing the outcome of the research from the outset. This kind of critical analysis is an aspect of the 'methodological imagination' about which we talked at the end of Chapter 1.

The other 'methods' question you would ask of any piece of research is to what population its conclusions are meant to generalize – of what is it supposed to be an example? Very little published research, even on single cases, is meant to illuminate just that single case. (In this respect it differs from the case-reports of the clinician or the social enquiry reports of the probation officer; these may be informed by the principles of research and, indeed, constitute a form of research, but they are seldom of sufficient general interest to be worth wider publication.) Where a single case is researched, it is often chosen as being typical of some class of cases or at least as casting light on some class of cases. Most research extends beyond the single case to the sample – large or small according to the type of design – which is to be taken as representative of a designated population. However, to take an obvious example, if all your research subjects are men then you would be unwise to generalize about 'the human race': women might be different. Quite a lot of research has based conclusions about a culture or even about people in general on research into white males – either students or volunteers – and neglected questions of gender, race, age, class/wealth, geographical location, degree of physical or mental impairment, and all the other characteristics which might have made a difference to the results if only they had been considered. In assessing a piece of research we often have to be aware of quite subtle ways in which a sample might appear typical of a given population, but can in fact be unrepresentative because of the way in which it has been selected. So another aspect of the 'methodological imagination' is that, if we are satisfied that the conclusions hold up for the case or the sample under consideration, we still have to think about the extent to which they also hold up for the wider population of which the case or sample is said to be representative or typical.

Having assessed whether the methods and arguments of the paper are valid, you will want to return, with more confidence, to the paper's contents. Research is ultimately about substance – about the problems and questions which it explores – and not about its methods. Taking into account any reservations to which we may have come as a result of your analysis of methods, what you will want to know is whether the paper tells you anything new and interesting. Does it add to or elucidate theory? Does it inform or criticize the operation of policy? Does it suggest anything which you can use to improve or modify your own professional practice?

Ethical and political questions

Finally, a further set of questions will also need to be considered as we build up an assessment of a piece of published research – Questions 6–9 on the check-list at the beginning of the chapter. Whether anyone was harmed or inconvenienced by the research is the basic 'minimum question' of research ethics: did the researchers act responsibly, to leave the world no worse a place by reason of their investigation? We may reasonably go on to ask whether there is any benefit to the 'subjects' or 'informants' of the research, and whether the research is justified if there is none. This means, for example, asking in whose interests the research was carried out. Is it obviously commissioned by management, for example, to look into how workers can best be exploited – or dominated by that perspective, even if not formally commissioned? Is it to do with the social control of working class people, or youths or women? Is it set up to explore how the convenience of doctors or nurses or hospitals can best be served? More fundamentally, we may ask whether the research paid proper attention to the fact that it was *people* who were involved in it. Some feminists (see, for example, Reinharz 1979) have likened conventional social research to the act of rape: a researcher goes in to a situation, takes out of it what he or she needs for his own ends (publication, academic esteem, promotion), and leaves the subjects/respondents/informants at best not much harmed; they certainly obtain no benefit from the process, but are used merely to satisfy the needs of the researcher.

These three questions do not affect the results, though they may affect our opinion of the researcher, but they lead quite naturally into a yet more fundamental one: does the way in which the research is framed embody ideological presuppositions such that the outcome is 'written in' or 'predetermined' by the original conceptual analysis and design? In other words, is there a very bad failure of the 'research imagination' in this research?

$$\equiv 3 \equiv$$

Reading open interviewing research

Exercise 10

This chapter is based around Section 2 of Abbot and Sapsford (1987b) *Community Care for Mentally Handicapped Children* – ' "Leaving it to Mum": motherhood and mental handicap'. If you can get hold of this, you might like to read through it quickly before proceeding. A slightly shortened version is reproduced in the Reader which is designed to accompany this volume – Abbott and Sapsford (1992) *Research into Practice: a reader for nurses and the caring professions*.

While reading, bear in mind the list of questions suggested at the beginning of Chapter 2; it will also form the basis of our comments below. (However, we shall not try to answer every one of the 10 questions for every one of the research papers on which we comment.) Also, make a list of the questions that you would have liked to ask us, if you had the opportunity, about how we did the research.

The research paper: Abbott and Sapsford (1987b)

This paper describes an interview study which we carried out in a new town in the middle 1980s, plus some data drawn from Abbott's earlier doctoral work (Abbott 1982). It is part of a longer monograph which also sets mental handicap in its historical context and traces the development of government policy towards people with learning difficulties. (These were most commonly called 'mentally handicapped people' at the time when it was written; terminology changes as sensitivity develops and as situations are re-theorized.) As you would expect, the paper starts with a brief exposition of the 'problem' and why it is interesting:

> The policy of 'community care' for mentally handicapped children has non-financial costs for families: work which in institutions would be wage-labour becomes unpaid work for 'Mum' when the burden of care is transferred to the family. This paper looks at the nature and extent of

such work and at the extent to which it alters the nature of the mother's life. We look also at the price which is paid by the whole family for the fact of having a mentally handicapped child . . . (The 'price' differs markedly from family to family, depending at least in part on the degree of handicap, the extent of associated physical handicaps and the social and economic situation of the family: what follows is a composite, not necessarily true to the experience of any one mother.)

(Abbott and Sapsford 1987b: 45–6)

We are reminded, right from the start, that even though this is detailed 'open' interviewing of a very small number of 'cases', nonetheless what is to be presented is an average or typification, with some idea of the range of variability around that average, and not straightforward life histories of particular mothers.

The method of the joint interview study is described thus:

Sixteen families were contacted from a list extracted for us from the school rolls of two Special Schools in the new city (one designated for the mildly handicapped and one for the severely). We carried out two interviews with each mother separated by about a year, not using a formal questionnaire but rather trying for the atmosphere of a friendly chat about life and work between neighbours. Although the interviews were tape-recorded, it seems to us that this atmosphere was readily attained in most cases . . . These data are contrasted with a parallel series of interviews with mothers of children who have *not* been labelled mentally handicapped.

(p. 46)

So we know that the method was 'open interviewing' cast in a 'life-history' mould – asking women to describe their current and past lives, but steering them towards topics of particular interest to the researchers. We note that the 'sample' is not statistically *representative* – one would not wish to say that because half or a quarter of the sample said or felt something, then half or a quarter of the corresponding population were likely to do so. However, it is a reasonably *typical* sample in the sense that it shows a reasonable range of cases, in terms both of the ages of the children, and of the degree and type of their condition, so any major problems (or any conspicuous lack of them) would probably be represented somewhere in it.

The account was written for a particular publication format, and its length had to be kept down, so many of the details which might have appeared have been omitted. The paper does not mention some of the strengths of the procedure. For example, we failed to record in the paper that we went in with an 'agenda' of basic questions which we wanted to cover somewhere in the interview. Though they were seldom or never asked explicitly, they served to make sure that key topics were covered by everyone, and that we did not form conclusions on the fact that someone had failed to talk about something important to us, when the fact of the matter was simply that it had failed to

come up in the conversation. Chief among the strengths was the sheer naturalism of the situation. The interviewers were very evidently a couple, having 'got
together' not all that long ago, and some of the atmosphere of a 'family visit'
was sometimes achieved; it is remarkably natural for one couple to be talking
to another mother about children and the experience of bringing them up.
Pamela's pregnancy helped here. By the time Pamela had been settled comfort-
ably in a chair and cushions arranged to support her, and Roger had been
taken to one side and asked how she liked her coffee (a curious variant on the
'Does she take sugar?' phenomenon), some degree of acquaintance seemed
already to have grown up. Later in the interview series some of the same effect
was unwittingly achieved by the small child we brought with us in a carrycot
for want of babysitting facilities.

Among what is not recorded is some of the detail of the informants, the
interviewing and how it progressed which might have helped the reader judge
its validity. The paper does not record, for instance, that the tape-recorder did
not work for the first interview, so that we were reduced to sitting down afterwards and writing out, independently, everything we could remember that
was said. It does not record the number of tapes which were difficult to
decipher afterwards because of the noise of children playing in the room or
building work going on outside. It does not talk about the interviews which
were difficult to 'get going', nor give much detail about the roles in which
informants tended to cast us and how these changed. We do not talk much
about the individual mothers, in fact, and this detracts from the richness of the
presentation.

One of the findings we report, as you might expect, is that the mothers to
whom we talked are very aware of their children's status as 'handicapped' and
very aware of other people's reactions to it. Apart from the obvious reactions
of strangers, even more difficult to deal with are the 'ignorant' reactions of
friends and neighbours:

> When I talk to people and I say 'Mark is mentally handicapped', and as
> soon as they know he is coming up to sixteen, you see, you know what I
> mean? . . . You see it before they even say it . . . It is an unspoken look
> . . . there is that fear of danger to 'my daughter'.

Such reactions can be looked for even from within the family:

> Let's put it this way, there were relations we have not seen since we found
> out about Trevor . . . [and] we have only been invited to tea with Trevor
> once to my brother-in-law. He thinks we should put Trevor away.

The mother's life comes very much to centre round the 'handicapped' child, in
a majority of cases. The amount of sheer physical labour – washing and
cleaning – is immense, with children who will normally not become 'house-
trained' till substantially after other children – in their teens or never, in the
most severe cases. Another part of the burden is constant supervision; as one
mother pointed out, you expect to have to be home to supervise a 5-year-old,
but not a 15-year-old. In many different ways these mothers' children caused

extra work and took up extra time, and the fact that the labour was freely and lovingly given did not diminish its extent. In all this it was clear that the concept of 'community care' basically meant 'care by mother'. Some had help from neighbours, some from immediate household, some from wider family, but in many cases the help was intermittent or trivial, and in many cases it did not occur. Eight of the sixteen families had no help from neighbours, and six of these also received little or no help from kin.

We also attempted a tentative typology of 'coping strategies' – trying to find a characterization of women's (or families') lives as a whole which would differentiate some families from others in terms of the general 'style' of their self-placement with regard to the outside world and some women from others in terms of the constructs they used to characterize and justify their lives. We noted a difference between those families which seemed determined that life should go on 'as normal' and those which conceded that there was something with which to 'cope'. Within the latter class we noted the 'bare copers' – those who managed from day to day and year to year – and those who seemed to have formed some stable kind of 'adaptation' to their situation. Within the latter class again we noted that some women seemed to have adopted the 'wife and/or mother' designation – seen as a positive role, not a form of constraint – as a preferred characterization of their current lives and as a description of their life goals. That is, they found themselves satisfied with what they were doing and appeared not to desire for any form of change.

We went on in this study – unusually for research into 'social problem' categories – to attempt a comparison with the 'normal':

> Shortly after the second interviews . . . one of us conducted a series of interviews with a 'sample' of mothers whose children had *not* been labelled as mentally handicapped, roughly matched for size of family and area of residence (which correlates well, in the new city, both with social class and with availability of 'social resource'). The sample is of course too small and haphazard to be representative of mothers in general . . . but the two samples match closely enough for some tentative conclusions to be drawn. One can after all say little about what is distinctive in the experience of mothering mentally handicapped children except by comparison with the general experience of mothering.
>
> (p. 65)

Overall we found similar kinds of work being done by the two samples, with a similar lack of help from both community and kin, but the work was greater in extent and more demanding for the mothers of children with learning difficulties, and they received even less help from kin and community.

The biggest difference between the two samples of families came in the kind of future that they could foresee. In the normal course of events children grow up and leave home, and women receive back their power to dispose of their daily time. Children with learning difficulties do not necessarily leave home unless the parents actively determine that they shall do so, and the feelings of guilt and apprehension which are associated with the child's teenage years colour the whole view of the future. For some families the decision will effectively be taken for them by events: one or two of the children were so severely physically handicapped that they were not expected to live into their twenties. For others it was clear that a decision would have to be taken, in the child's interests. Some families were adamant that their child would stay with them, for ever if need be:

> When you think what her mental age is, say four or five, by the time she's nineteen she won't be more than that. You wouldn't stick a five year old in a hostel, would you?

(p. 74)

For many, however, the decision is a mixture of the child's interests, the convenience of the family and a feeling that in some way the problems of an adult 'child' are beyond what the neighbourhood can cope with.

Finally, the paper summarizes the study's conclusions about

> . . . the real cost of bearing and bringing up a mentally handicapped child in the community. Some of it – the day to day grind of 'child work' – falls largely on the child's mother . . . The rearing of a mentally handicapped baby does not differ in kind from the rearing of any other baby – itself a substantial social burden – but it differs in its density and its duration . . . The burden goes on, moreover, potentially for ever, unless the decision is made to send the child away . . . Specific to mental handicap . . . are the other range of major problems which families encounter: the reactions . . . among strangers and also within the family and kin group.

(pp. 74–5)

Discussion

In what purports to be an evaluation of research methods we have spent a fair amount of time looking at the substantive findings of the study – what it has to say about mothering children with learning difficulties. We have also given you additional information which was not in the report but which might be thought vital if the research is to be properly evaluated. This will not, of course, be possible when we are discussing the research of others. We cannot generally, when reading a report, ask researchers questions which might provide additional information about their methods and methodologies. It is therefore important, when writing up research, to consider what material about the methods has to be included to answer possible questions. Limitations of space often cause problems, however, and researchers often respond to them by leaving out the information which is vital for an informed evaluation of the research.

We read research studies mostly to look at what they have found out, not to study their methods. The study of methods comes in, however, when we need to determine whether we believe what is stated, whether it accords with the evidence as given, and whether the conclusions are possible ones given the ways in which the data have been collected. We need to look then to the strengths of each method, in general and in the particular case under examination, and to the corresponding weaknesses of logic of that type of research in general or this particular example of it.

One very definite strength of 'open' approaches to research – just talking to people, or observing and participating in their lives (discussed in the next chapter), without imposing much structure on what is collected – is the immediacy, the vivacity, the feeling of actually 'being there'. The Abbott and Sapsford piece carries the actual words of the informants and lets them tell their own stories, often better than we could tell them for them. No amount of second-hand description can convey what it may be like to have a mentally handicapped child nearly as powerfully as the words of Mrs Miller:

> For about a month after I found out I didn't have any feeling for her any way – she wasn't my baby, she was just *a* baby that had got to be looked after and fed and kept clean . . . [And then] I walked past the pram one day and she looked up at me and she smiled at me . . . she just smiled . . . After that I was all right.
>
> (p. 47)

The price that is paid for this power and immediacy, which comes from the detailed study of a few cases or a single setting, is a necessary doubt about the representative nature of the 'sample'. To what extent does an interview study of less than 20 mothers of mentally handicapped children in one geographical location tell us anything about the problems nationwide of this kind of community care? In our study we did our best to 'cover the range' – to include as wide a range of 'cases' and social settings as was possible. We sampled, for instance, mothers from both a 'severe' school and a 'mild' school, so we could reasonably expect to contact cases ranging from near-total physical and mental inability to children who could have passed for 'just a bit stupid' at ordinary schools (and we did, in fact, contact cases covering this entire range). Our sample was well scattered through a new city in which geographical locality is fairly well correlated with social class and material circumstances, and we had everything from a mother permanently on social security to one in a substantial rural house set in its own grounds. Some of the sample were 'immigrants' of recent date to the new town, some had moved there in the 1940s and 1950s from London, and some were locally born and still to a large part involved in the original local 'village' community. However, we do not know how representative the new city is of places where parents whose children have learning difficulties might be living. Thus, even if we are fairly confident that the results generalize to all families with a child with learning difficulties in that city, we would probably be less confident that they would generalize to families living in other parts of the country. Also, we do not know the extent to which looking after a child with learning difficulties is typical of caring for other groups of dependents.

We would certainly not want to assert that a particular percentage of all such mothers held this or that belief, or experienced this or that problem, on the basis of our handful of cases, but the problems experienced by our informants are probably not far different from those experienced by all such mothers. Nonetheless, all were 'customers' of the same schools and health and social service provision, so a study carried out elsewhere might well come up with different experiences depending on how much service differs across the country. Our study was also tied to a particular historical time, since which there have been major changes: we do not know how the newer policy of integrating mentally handicapped children into the 'normal' schools has affected the lives of mothers.

The other question which must be asked of this kind of research, where so much depends on the building of relationships and so much is apparently 'left in the hands of the informants', is the extent to which the findings are specific to those particular relationships, or even 'created' by something that the researchers did or said. The only guard against this, and the only warrant of validity, is constant reflexivity in the research and in the report of it – constant attention paid to what is going on, and detailed discussion of all aspects of the social situation and the procedures in the report. Our report is weak in this respect; it is characteristic of short reports of 'open' research that what is omitted in order to keep length down is the reflexive account, important as it is, and while reflexive material has been supplied, there is not as much of it here as we would have liked.

One aspect of reflexivity which you should look for in research reports is an awareness of the crucial importance of role and audience in the construction of interview data. 'What is expected' differs according to setting: the accounts we give when we are 'doing a public performance' are different from those we might produce in the privacy of the home. Similarly, a male interviewer may be faced with a different kind of account from what would be produced for a female, and the same goes for young *v.* old, black *v.* white, able-bodied *v.* disabled . . . The account which we produce is very much conditioned by who we see the interviewer as being and, therefore, what is to be seen as 'relevant' or 'useful'.

Informants *have* to make sense of the situation before they can function within it, and how they do so is much conditioned by what we present the situation as being. They have to use the clues we provide to work out what we are after and what we shall see as relevant. One common way of introducing this kind of research task, for instance, is to present it as one which a student has to do as a requirement of the degree. The risk here is that to present the interviews as just something that a student has to do may devalue the task and lead the informants to produce accounts which are easy, memorable and picturesque, but not necessarily 'true' in any usual sense. The major alternative tack is to present the work as 'research', as in the Abbott and Sapsford study, but the problem here is that the term 'research' is ambiguous in common language and has no single clear meaning. Our informants were quite clear as to why they were being interviewed: they knew they had been approached because their children had learning difficulties. Most started off by identifying us with some branch of the support services – as doctors, psychologists, social workers – and assuming that we were in some way checking up on the efficiency of provision. When they realized that these identifications did not hold up, we tended to 'become' the other kind of researcher – people writing a book and looking for useful material. (The mothers knew they had a story worth telling.) When this role transition took place, the nature of the accounts tended to change. The informants became more relaxed. The conversation became more general and it was easier to probe for detail not immediately relevant to the question of mental handicap. On the other hand, the informants were often less precise and less analytic in stating what they had experienced and what they felt they needed.

A problem with accounts, which you need to look out for in evaluating published research of this kind, is that we all have many different ways of accounting for ourselves, many different stories to tell. There are, for instance, public 'rhetorics' which people tend to produce in a rounded, 'rehearsed' form when asked direct questions. Some of them are minimal, polite, 'safe', problem-avoiding accounts such as Cornwell (1984) calls 'public accounts' – something uncontroversial which is always safe to produce when questioned on this topic. Others are learned rhetorics: the first response on the subject of social class from anyone who has studied sociology, for instance, tends to recapitulate some part of the course studied. Others again are 'class-markers' – to state certain kinds of beliefs communicates membership of a class or group, or sympathy with it. Others again are just well rehearsed stories, polished and perhaps partly falsified or simplified by frequent telling. All or any of these rhetorics may truly be held as beliefs by the informant, and any or all *may* be acted out in practice, but the chances are that they are sincerely held, but purely verbal beliefs, unconnected in any way to action. One always strives to get 'underneath' these rhetorics, to get the informant analysing his or her own life in a fresh way and producing 'true' accounts. However, one should note that these 'private' accounts are equally a product of a particular social situation – the informant striving to make sense of his or her life in the light of his or her perception of what is relevant and useful for the interviewer – so we cannot treat these as necessarily 'more true' than the rhetorics and polished stories.

The points which are important here as guidelines for the evaluation of research are:

1 that informants do not 'give interviewers the facts', but work out the purpose of the interview and give accounts that will make sense and be relevant in the context of that purpose;
2 that they are constrained by what they think is acceptable (as well as relevant) to say to different kinds of people, in different kinds of tasks;
3 that we all have accounts of common topics which 'roll easily off the tongue', but we may have other and possibly contradictory things to say about them if one can get behind the rhetoric; and
4 that any given account may be a rhetoric in this sense, but nonetheless not

'rhetorical' – well practised verbal accounts may or may not be accurate descriptions of behaviour and attitudes.

You would expect to find enough reflexive material in a good account of open interviewing to enable you to form some view on these questions: whether the situation partly dictated the response, whether the interviewer has taken a rhetoric for a reality, whether a well practised account, nonetheless, describes a reality of the informant's lives. To the extent that such material is not present, you may have to suspend judgement on the credibility of the results – not necessarily to disbelieve them, but to give them less credit than if their validity was well established.

A second question when evaluating the scope of a piece of research – the opposite of the question of how far it can be generalized – is how *specific* the findings are. In the Abbott and Sapsford paper one important question was the extent to which the experiences of those who care for children with learning difficulties are *different* from those of other mothers (all mothering being, in a sense, a form of community care). For this reason we also interviewed a group of mothers whose children had *not* been labelled as having learning difficulties and so were able to distinguish the problems of having children with learning difficulties from the problems of having children in general. (Naturally we took pains to pick a comparison group as like the mothers of children with learning difficulties as possible, so that where differences were found they were not equally likely to be due to age or class/material circumstances or area of residence.)

It is worth noting that the interviews with the mothers whose children were not labelled as having learning difficulties were far more difficult than those with mothers whose children were so labelled. The mothers of children with learning difficulties 'knew' what they were being interviewed about – they knew that what we had picked out was mothers in their situation. The other mothers had far more difficulty making sense of the situation. There was no obvious 'social problem' which we might be investigating, and they could not see what it was about their situation which made it interesting for us to get them to 'tell their story'. They therefore had great difficulty working out what story to tell. As we said above, the sense which the informant makes of the situation is a key determinant of the accounts which are elicited in interview.

Summary: points for evaluation

1 When reading 'open interview' research, you need to know quite a lot about the interviewer, the situation and the course of the interviews, to judge the validity of the results. *Reactivity* – the production of material in response to loaded questions, or the reshaping of it to suit the expected prejudices of the interviewer – is a particularly strong possibility in this kind of research.

2 One might be suspicious of research reports based on one quick interview with each informant; the likelihood of the interviewer getting beyond the

'rhetoric' or 'public account' is not high (see Cornwell 1984, particularly p. 16).

3 At a more subtle level, you need to work out what sense the informants probably made of the situation, in order to see what they will have perceived as relevant and what they may have omitted or ignored in their accounts.

4 To the extent that there is insufficient reflexive material for you to make these judgements, you do not need to reject the research report entirely, but its conclusions should be handled with some caution.

5 Looking at the 'sample' you should ask yourself how far the results are likely to generalize beyond the immediate informants – of what are these informants typical?

6 You should also ask yourself how specific the results are to the type of person or setting which is being described – to what extent they might be equally true of quite different groups or settings.

Exercise 11

Now re-read the Abbott and Sapsford paper in the light of this chapter, bearing in mind the points listed at the end. Note particularly how much extra material we have had to supply in this chapter in order to give you any real insight into the process of the interviews and the ways in which we were typecast by informants. Look back at the questions you thought you would have liked to ask us. How many of them have been answered by the 'extra' material we have provided in this chapter?

Further reading

On children with learning difficulties

Abbott, Pamela and Sapsford, Roger (1986). 'Diverse reports: caring for mentally handicapped children in the community' *Nursing Times*, 5 March, 47–9.

Bayley, M. (1973). *Mental Handicap and Community Care.* London: Routledge and Kegan Paul.

Glendinning, C. (1983). *Unshared Care: Parents and their Disabled Children.* London: Routledge and Kegan Paul.

Shearer, A. (1972). *A Report on Public and Professional Attitudes towards the Sexual and Emotional Attitudes of Handicapped People.* London: Spastics Society/ National Association for Mental Handicap.

Voysey, M. (1975). *A Constant Burden: The Reconstitution of Family Life.* London: Routledge and Kegan Paul.

On 'normal' mothering

Abbott, Pamela and Wallace, Claire (1990). *An Introduction to Sociology: Feminist Perspectives.* London: Routledge and Kegan Paul.

Backett, K. (1982). *Mothers and Fathers.* London: Macmillan.

Boulton, M. (1983). *On Being a Mother.* London: Tavistock.

Kitzinger, S. (1978). *Women as Mothers*. London: Fontana.
Oakley, A. (1972). *Sex, Gender and Society*. London: Fontana.
Porter, M. (1983). *Home, Work and Class Consciousness*. Manchester: Manchester University Press.

On coping and coping strategies

Davis, F. (1963). *Passage through Crisis: Polio Victims and their Families*. Indianapolis: Bobbs-Merril.
Goffman, E. (1961). *Asylums: Essays on the Social Situation of Mental Patients and other Inmates*. Harmondsworth: Penguin.
Goffman, E. (1963). *Stigma: The Management of Spoilt Identities*. Harmondsworth: Penguin.
Roth, J. (1963). *Timetables*. Indianapolis: Bobbs-Merril.

Reading observation research

This Chapter deals with interpretative observation studies which involve varying degrees of participation; 'systematic' observation is dealt with under the heading of survey research. The chapter is built around three research papers.

Mavis Kirkham (1983). 'Labouring in the dark', in J. Wilson-Barnett (ed.) *Nursing Research: Ten Studies in Patient Care*, published by Wiley, Chichester.

Jean Orr (1986). 'Working with women's health groups', in A. While (ed.) *Research in Preventive Community Nursing: Fifteen Studies in Health Visiting*, also published by Wiley, Chichester.

Nicky James (1984). 'A postscript to nursing', in C. Bell and H. Roberts (eds) *Sociological Research: Politics, Problems, Practice*, published by Routledge and Kegan Paul, London.

All three are reprinted in slightly shortened form in Abbott and Sapsford (1992), the Reader associated with this text.

Exercise 12

Now would be a good time to read the first of these three, the paper by Mavis Kirkham, 'Labouring in the dark'.

Research Paper 1: Kirkham (1983)

Mavis Kirkham's paper deals with the event of giving birth in hospital and the time leading up to it. Her focus of interest is the transmission – or non-transmission – of information from doctors, nurses and midwives to the pregnant woman, about the progress of her imminent delivery and the timescale that may be expected. She is interested in the hierarchical relationship between nurses and midwives, and patients, and the way in which this may, in fact, impede delivery by failing to reassure patients and not allowing them to draw on their own strengths during the process.

What she did was to sit in on 90 labours in one consultant unit of a northern teaching hospital, take notes of what was said and done and talk to the women after their babies had been born; she also talked to 85 patients in hospital before confinement. In addition, she observed five home confinements and 18 confinements in a neighbouring GP unit, and she interviewed a number of midwives. Her method was that of open, unstructured, participant observation:

> I wanted to see what issues were important to those involved as shown in their actions and words at the time. Observation was clearly an appropriate method . . . I came to this research as a midwife and a mother. But my observations were guided by those aspects of care in labour which the midwives and mothers I observed showed were important to them. Thus my observations and analysis were 'grounded' (Glaser and Strauss 1967) in the experiences of those observed as shown in their words and actions.
>
> (Kirkham 1983: 86)

The aim is to describe not necessarily a fully representative sample of confinements, but at least a sample of typical ones:

> These labours were chosen as normal labours, as far as anyone can tell this in advance. I therefore did not observe women with known medical or obstetric abnormalities.
>
> (p. 86)

Kirkham describes and illustrates the main tactics she sees the pregnant women using in order to get information. Straightforward questions are, of course, asked, but this is not always a good tactic for gaining information – questions are often deflected or blocked 'in the patient's interests' or 'because she wouldn't really understand'. Another tactic is to make what appears to be a statement, but which has the force of a question – for example:

> *Patient*: My backside's hurting. It'll be the cut. [Silence] . . . It's the episiotomy.
> *Sister*: It's not an episiotomy. It's a tear. But it hasn't gone anywhere it shouldn't.
>
> (p. 90)

Some patients try out statements in the form of jokes:

> *Patient*: Is there much water?
> *Doctor*: A normal amount.
> *Patient*: You imagine buckets!
> *Doctor*: You've not got that much when you get to term . . .
>
> (p. 90)

Some combine this with what Kirkham calls 'self-denigration':

> *Student midwife*: Let's see if the machine is playing silly beggars. (Patient
> pulls up her gown to show the . . . connection to the monitor.)
> *SM*: You're a right flasher, aren't you?
> *Patient*: And I've got such a wonderful body. (Both laugh. SM listens to
> fetal heart. Patient asks if she can listen. SM lets her . . .)
>
> (p. 91)

Passive watching and the active drawing of conclusions is a common tactic
here as elsewhere – 'If it was going to be quick they wouldn't have given me
Pethidine' – but it is limited by the extent to which what is seen is correctly
understood. A certain amount can be gleaned from eavesdropping on teaching
sessions, where sisters are instructing student midwives, for instance, but this
essentially passive tactic does not lend itself to gaining useful – usable and
interpretable – information.

All of this is contrasted with deliveries in GP units and at home. On the GP
units, not surrounded by senior medical staff, midwives were freer with information and found it necessary to solicit the patient's co-operation more.
Patients delivered at home tended to *demand* to know what was going on.

The author concludes that the women on the ward want and need information with which to orient themselves within the process of birth, and that what
they receive is generally inadequate. The lack of information very much con-
strains their choices. A hierarchy of relations, and of control of information,
runs from the patient at the bottom through midwives and sisters to doctors.
Kirkham observes that the tactics which patients use to elicit information from
midwives run remarkably parallel to those which midwives use to elicit information from doctors. She comments in conclusion that an awareness of problems *shared* by midwife and patient could do much to change midwives'
behaviour, which in turn could fundamentally change the patient's experience
of labour.

Exercise 13

Now read Jean Orr (1986) 'Working with women's health groups: the community
health movement'.

Research Paper 2: Orr (1986)

This paper describes some of Jean Orr's experiences and observations while
working with women's health groups.

> Over a period of three years I have been involved in working with ten
> women's health groups in the north-west of England. I came to work
> with these groups as part of ongoing research into well women clinics

and my concern about women's health. This work was, and is, largely an expression of my belief in feminism and from this ensued a commitment to share whatever skills I had with other women . . . research was an outcome of my involvement, not a reason for it. Nurses and health visitors are in a key position to assist women achieve optimum health, but only if they listen to what women are saying. These groups provided an opportunity to listen to women who were concerned about health but were not likely to make these concerns known to professionals.

(Orr 1986: 192)

This might be seen as 'action research': a facility is set up or a change is made, with the researcher involved in the process, and the report describes what happened. Typically (though not inevitably), the research technique is one of participant observation – being a participant, the researcher takes notes on what he or she personally experiences. Orr's research was of this kind:

I was a participant observer of these groups. The theoretical rationale for the use of participant observation is based on three concepts. Firstly, the basic . . . perspective of attempting to understand social facts in their wider context encourages the observation of the total life of a community . . . rather than the abstraction of selected variables. Secondly, the need to define how various social actors in a given context perceive their situation [implies] . . . that what people believe to be is as significant as that which is. Thirdly . . . the phenomena being studied are undergoing continuous change . . .

(pp. 192–3)

The driving force behind what she does, in one sense, is feminist-informed professional practice – making her skills and knowledge available to women in as non-authoritarian a form as possible. In another, the driving force is political: 'I was concerned with making these women's experiences visible and influential in effecting changes in health care provision.' (p. 192).

The mode of operation of the groups varied. The content of the session often bore only a derived relationship to what was advertised, as the conversation led away from the specific to more general preoccupations – 'contraception' developed into a discussion of female sexuality, and 'motherhood' into a discussion of women's role in the family and experiences of 'domestic violence'. That for many women this was their first opportunity to share their feelings on topics such as these and to discover that their experiences were not unique was very apparent, as was the pain and discomfort sometimes involved in looking at such personal and heavily defended topics in an analytic way.

Orr's overall conclusions are, firstly, that throughout the groups the women had achieved only marginal involvement with the health services and had experienced severe crises to do with the social aspects of health problems, crises which the health services had not managed to ameliorate. They needed to come together informally, as women, to share experiences and learn from each other, rather than to be 'placed under the rule of an expert'. Her second conclusion, for the practice of health visiting, was about the useful information which health visitors could glean from feminist writings about common female experiences. Finally, she stresses the importance of informal groups such as those she has studied, and their potential for delivering a part of the service for which health visitors see themselves as being responsible.

Research Paper 3: James (1984)

These previous articles have both been short papers, and what is conspicuously missing is any great degree of reflexivity. In Jean Orr's paper, for example, we might have expected to find some discussion of how the fact that she was running the groups might have affected what she found; her control of the topic of conversation, and presumably of its timing and routing as well, would put her in a strong position to direct the outcome – perhaps unknowingly, guiding the conversation in certain directions and even eliciting certain emotional responses without realizing the degree of control which she was exerting. (We do not say that she *did* do so, but only that the possibility cannot be ruled out on the basis of this report.) We do not even know whether she told the group members that she might be writing up her experiences as a research paper – which might be seen as an important ethical question. Mavis Kirkham is more explicit about how her position may have affected the behaviour of the women she observed:

> I sat during most of the labours level with the patient's head about six feet from her and took constant written notes. The question of the researcher's influence upon the research is raised by this method . . . The people I observed may well have been on their 'best behaviour' because I was observing them.
>
> (Kirkham 1983: p. 86)

We know from the last chapter, however, that there is more than the discussion of reactivity to a proper reflexive account. How the researcher is received and what sense the participants make of her are part of the story that needs to be told. We also need, however, to know more about the researcher herself, her theoretical perspectives, her professional expectations – anything which may affect the conduct of the research or the interpretation of the data.

The third paper to be considered in this chapter, Nicky James' 'A postscript to nursing', is not a report of research results, but an extended reflexive account, written for a book of articles on the research process. James describes what it was like, as a trained nurse, to return to the wards to do research on nursing for a higher degree. It raises many of the special problems (and the strengths) of the open participation method in an acute form.

Exercise 14

You might like to read the paper at this point: Nicky James (1984) 'A postscript to nursing'.

James went in 'labelled' as a researcher and had no role into which she could 'disappear from view'. Whether participant research should be open or covert (secret) is much debated. Covert research obviously disturbs what is going on less; if the researcher can pass as a natural member of the scene, then there is no 'researcher identity' to which participants might react. This obviously holds even more where the researcher *is* a natural participant in the context, e.g. Jean Orr running the women's groups about which she wants to write. (There are problems of detachment here, however; it is very difficult to stand back from your own real-life involvement.) The disadvantage of covert research is that you tend to be 'stuck' in one part of the field and bound by the limitations of the adopted role: if you have 'become' a nurse, then you cannot also socialize with doctors on equal terms and experience what the patients experience. You are also limited in the number and type of questions you can ask about what is going on before you start looking unnaturally incompetent and ignorant for a true participant. Some might also consider covert research unethical, in that participants are deceived into revealing things about themselves which they might not have chosen to reveal to a researcher and an abuse of relationships is involved.

Open research has the converse disadvantage, that participants have to make sense of you and will generally try to consider what they do and say because they know it may be recorded. The presence of an explicit researcher may also be uncomfortable for the other participants because it forces them to question aspects of their behaviour which are normally taken for granted and may partially destroy the careful set of 'cognitive defences' which we all set up against the unpleasant or boring aspects of our jobs and our lives in general. To the extent that real involvement is achieved, moreover, the researcher will also acquire some of these defences, and breaking through them into analysis will become a real emotional problem. (This is also a problem for covert researchers, of course – sometimes more so.) James certainly found both problems during her research relationships with other nurses:

> A dysfunction built into the research . . . was the constant prodding at the defence mechanisms which are a means of continuing at the unit. If I pushed the others too far they would evade, avoid or tell me to shut up, but my own defences were also under scrutiny and the more I was per-turbed by exposing them, the more my reluctance to write up at the end of the day grew. I was enjoying the nursing. For the research, philosophy, the structure of the National Health Service, and numbers became easier lines of thought. None of them had anything to do with people.
>
> (James 1984: 141–2)

One of the major problems of undertaking fieldwork, particularly in the role of 'the researcher', is to establish a role within the setting which is something other than sitting and taking notes. As a qualified nurse, Nicky James found it particularly difficult to be present on a ward for which she had no nursing responsibilities, as her fieldnotes show:

> I didn't know what I was doing, and the lack of routine was very undermining, or rather the lack of knowledge of the routine . . . I felt that I had no independence on the ward because I nearly always had to ask people if I wanted to do, or thought I ought to do, something.
>
> (pp. 136–7)

> Confusion and doubt is part of any nurse's move to a new ward, but I had forgotten that and I found it difficult to make sense of things as a nurse, let alone a researcher.
>
> (p. 137)

Having acquired a role within the ward, she found it almost equally difficult to dissociate herself from it again.

The problem for the participants is making sense of the researcher and assigning her a social role, and some of the solutions may not always be flattering or even useful, as James points out:

> Nicky, you're sort of like a PS in a letter. Not part of the main body of the nursing team, but still important. (Night nurse)

> This is our pet sociologist, who's working on the unit and studying us. She's found out all sorts of interesting things. (Continuing care unit sister)
>
> (p. 129)

What sense will be made is essentially unpredictable, so one has to be prepared to make changes 'on the run'. James had this problem right from the start, in her initial discussions with 'gate-keepers':

> In the proposal to the nursing administrators, submitted before I went to see them, I tried to 'sell' myself by predicting what they would like . . . my main doubt was whether they would tolerate an observer. Why should they? To try to overcome that, I made a commitment to working free, instead of being an onlooker . . . I had totally misjudged their reading of the proposal. Instead of being flexible, it looked as though I did not know what I was doing, and though they welcomed nursing research, there was some anxiety over someone who wanted to be integrated . . . I acquiesced to their suggestions . . . In the report on the meeting I noted that 'I went in optimistic and came out feeling like a grilled sardine – small, squashed and hot.'
>
> (pp. 133–4)

In conclusion, James' account of her research reinforces very strongly the importance of reflexivity. She describes how difficult it was to 'get in' with any freedom of movement, how difficult it was to find herself a role which was plausible to herself, and how difficult it was for others to find a place for her in their social world. She makes it clear that observing was not a neutral process, but one which trampled over her own preconceptions and led to considerable emotional turmoil, the more so because her investigations also tended to trample over the preconceptions and defences of others.

Summary: points for evaluation

1 Observation research, like open interviewing, needs to show a substantial reflexive element in the report if we are able to judge the effect of researcher and situation on the recorded data, and how the way in which both researcher and participants make sense of the situation conditions what is produced.
2 In observation research even more than in open interviewing we need to know something of the researcher and his or her preconceptions, fears and capabilities, to put faith in the reported interpretations of the situation.
3 In covert research we need to know what kind of role the researcher took up, how convincing he or she was, and the extent to which the role may have tied him or her down to one segment or aspect of the situation and perhaps blinded him or her to interpretations which might seem valid from a different perspective.
4 In research where the researcher is a 'real' participant, carrying out his or her normal role as well as writing about the situation, we need to consider the extent to which it has been possible for him or her to step outside the professional assumptions of that situation for the purposes of the research analysis.

Exercise 15:

Now re-read the papers by Kirkham and Orr in the light of the James paper and our discussion.

Further reading

On maternity nursing

Cartwright, A. (1979). *The Dignity of Labour?* London: Tavistock.
Lorenson, Margarethe (1983). 'Effects of touch in patients during a crisis situation in hospital', in J. Wilson-Barnett (ed.) *Nursing Research: Ten Studies in Patient Care.* Chichester: Wiley.
Maternity Services Advisory Committee (1984). *Maternity Care in Action Pt II: Care during Childbirth.* London: HMSO.
Maternity Services Advisory Committee (1985). *Maternity Care in Action Pt III: Care of the Mother and Baby.* London: HMSO.
Metcalf, Clare (1983). 'A study of change in the method of organising the delivery of

nursing care in a ward of a maternity hospital', in J. Wilson-Barnett (ed.) op. cit.

Oakley, Ann (1980). *Women Confined: Towards a Sociology of Childbirth*. Oxford: Martin Robertson.

Oakley, Ann (1981). *From Here to Maternity*. Harmondsworth: Penguin.

Savage, Wendy (1986). *A Savage Enquiry: Who Controls Childbirth?* London: Virago.

Women's groups and health education

Dominelli, Lena and McLeod, Eileen (1989). *Feminist Social Work*. London: Macmillan.

Kenner, Charmian (1985). *No Time for Women: Exploring Women's Health in the 1930s and Today*. London: Pandora (particularly Chapter 4: 'Health education: laying the blame on women').

Sherlock, Effie (1987). 'The Liverpool experience: the Croxteth Women's Health Group – self-help on a deprived community of Liverpool', in J. Orr (ed.) *Women's Health in the Community*. Chichester: Wiley.

Williams, Anne (1987). 'Making sense of feminist contributions to women's health', also in the Orr volume.

Research on general ward nursing

Brown, Roswyn (1989). *Individualised Care: The Role of the Ward Sister*. Harrow: Scutari.

Cope, David (1981). *Organisational Development and Action Research in Hospitals*. Aldershot: Gower.

Wilson-Barnet Jenifer and Robinson, Sarah (eds) (1989). *Directions in Nursing Research*. Harrow: Scutari.

≡ 5 ≡

Reading about controlled trials

At the other extreme of the spectrum of research from open interviewing and observation comes the *controlled trial* or *experiment*. The central principle here is not finding out about the unknown, but testing known principles. The medical controlled trial tests the efficacy of a drug or treatment by applying the drug to one group of people and withholding it from another. To the extent that the first group are *exactly* like the second in terms of personal characteristics and histories, and to the extent that they receive *exactly* the same treatment in all ways except that the drug is administered to the experimental group and withheld from the control group, then logically any difference between the two which is present at the end but was not present at the start must be due to the administration of the drug. The four essentials are: a clearly defined 'treatment'; a clearly defined 'outcome'; a comparison of outcomes between treatment and non-treatment, or between different treatments; and control of anything else which might otherwise have explained observed differences in outcome.

Generally, we associate experimental research with highly scientific subject-areas – medicine, the more scientific kinds of psychology, etc. It is quite possible, however, to apply precisely the same principles to much more 'woolly' topic areas, such as the treatment of mental conditions, and the first paper considered in this chapter is the evaluation of an experimental nurse-administered treatment for women's depression – Verona Gordon's 'Treatment of depressed women by nurses in Britain'.

Exercise 16

You might now like to read the paper by Verona Gordon (1986). The full text, entitled 'Treatment of depressed women by nurses in Britain and the USA', can be found in Julia Brooking (ed.) *Psychiatric Nursing Research*, published by Wiley. A shortened version which omits the USA material will be found in Abbott and Sapsford (1992).

Research Paper 1: Gordon (1986)

Verona Gordon's paper begins with a discussion of the extent to which depression can be considered one of the major health problems of women. Twice as many women as men are diagnosed depressed around the world and the incidence of the condition shows an alarming growth over time. (Whether an increased incidence of *diagnosis* of depression over time necessarily equates with an increased *incidence* of depression is questionable, however. We shall return to this point in a later chapter.)

Gordon suggests that current treatment practices are not satisfactory for women's depression:

> There are two concerns that remain with treatment and prevention issues. One is that traditional treatment approaches by male therapists perpetuate the passivity and negative self-image of women . . . The other is that while there are numerous programmes to treat depression, treatment usually begins after the depression has reached a serious level. This lack of early identification and intervention does not support nursing's commitment to prevention and health maintenance.
>
> (Gordon 1986: 95)

She suggests that a group approach is far superior to individual therapy for women, in that it allows for peer support and gives a safe and rewarding environment within which negative self-labelling can be unlearned. The (female) professional nurse, she suggests, is uniquely well placed to run such groups successfully; she is herself a woman (though possibly better educated than some of those she serves), she appreciates the problems of women's positions and the value to them of both family and work, she is not seen by the public as having a judgmental or diagnostic role, and she is popularly stereotyped as someone who cares and offers support.

This paper reports on an experimental treatment group for women's depression which Gordon set up in England. (Two earlier studies were carried out in the United States – see Gordon 1982; Gordon and Ledray 1984).

> Twenty women, 40 to 60 years of age, were selected for the study. These subjects had been recruited through a public service radio broadcast (BBC airwaves) seeking depressed women as participants . . . There was an overwhelming response to the broadcast from hundreds of women . . . The University of London's phone lines were flooded with calls, confirming the author's belief that depression in women is extensive.
>
> (p. 100)

'Information meetings' were set up, at which 119 women who showed interest and met the criteria filled out a descriptive questionnaire and took two standardized tests of depression and suicidal pathology. Eighty-one women showed up on these tests as mildly to moderately depressed, and 20 of these were randomly selected for the treatment group. A similar-sized group of women were selected from the 81 as a control group, and they filled in the same tests as these 20 at around the same time. However,

. . . women assigned to the control condition received no intervention between pre-and post-testing. At the first information meeting they had been asked to refrain from joining other therapy groups or seeking counselling while the study was going on unless necessary.

(p. 105)

(The women who were not to be used in the study were, nonetheless, informed of their test results by post. Gordon telephoned the six who showed up as *very* depressed; all of them agreed to consult their GP.)

Meetings were arranged for the 20 women in a comfortable central location in London, and the discussion group began to meet. In the first meetings all the women were encouraged to 'tell their story', but subsequently such working over past ground was discouraged. Instead, a topic was assigned for each meeting – signs and symptoms of depression, assertiveness, goal-setting, conflict management, etc. – and this was discussed, with Gordon introducing educational material into the discussion. Homework tasks were set and a workbook issued. At the start of the series of meetings, all subjects filled in five self-report tests, all of proven reliability and widely used in research, covering self-esteem, social adjustment, loneliness, depression/hopelessness and 'life events' occurring. The same tests were re-administered at the end of the 14 group sessions.

The results were fairly clear-cut. There were no significant pre-treatment differences between the experimental group and the controls. Three of the tests – depression, self-esteem and hopelessness – showed significant post-test differences between the experimental group and the control group. *Prima facie* the results suggest strongly that the treatment made a difference to the attitudes and internal states of those who received it.

The author's conclusions are:

1 that professional nurses . . . tend to be effective facilitators of depressed women's groups;
2 that coping strategies for women can be taught, tested and shared within a supportive group atmosphere;
3 that replication of the intervention model with increased numbers of women of a variety of ages and backgrounds could be useful future nursing research.

The significance of the intervention model is:

1 to help women cope effectively, take an active role in their own health;
2 to prevent possible severe depression in women;
3 to gain data about the complex phenomena of depression in women;
4 to strengthen the family unit by increasing self-esteem of women.

(pp. 112–13)

(The first conclusion is possibly stronger than the design of the study warrants: one may not conclude that 'nurses tend' on the basis of results from one or a few nurses. The best that can be said is that nurses *are able to* act as facilitators.)

As an example of a 'controlled trial', this experiment in therapy shows many of the classic features of the true experiment as used in medicine or psychology, but falls down in some respects and is questionable in others. (This is not a criticism of the particular study, but the general verdict on the use of this research approach to evaluate events which happen outside the 'pure science' laboratory.) Its strength is in the clean lines of its design – a treatment applied to one group and withheld from another, with demonstrably little pre-treatment difference between the groups and demonstrably significant differences after the treatment. (The concept of 'significance' will be dealt with in a later chapter. For now, accept as a suitable simplification that a result is described as 'significant' if the odds against it occurring by chance are very high.)

There are two questions which might sensibly be asked of this as an experiment, however, issues on which it perhaps fails to reach the rigor of the 'true' laboratory experiment or hospital controlled trial.

1 The 'manipulation' is somewhat vaguely defined. If someone were to try to duplicate the procedures and obtained the opposite effect we would not know whether this argued against Gordon's findings or merely demonstrated that the new researcher had not, in fact, managed to duplicate Gordon's procedures. This is a general point about the evaluation of therapies.
2 The second potential criticism concerns the measure of outcome – the questionnaires which the subjects filled in. At least in this study we have what purports to be an objective measure of outcome – as opposed to therapist's or patient's judgement, which are obviously suspect in this context. However, this fact that the 'measures' are predesigned questionnaires purporting to give a score for some predetermined mental trait, state or circumstance is always a reason for pausing to think about the research. We shall discuss such measures in the next chapter and elsewhere in the book. You might want to ask yourself, however, the extent to which you could realistically expect any kind of prestructured questionnaire to reflect people's real experience of the complex, social phenomenon which we call depression. (Note, however, that this criticism does not necessarily hold true for the test used to select the experimental and control groups. These did not purport to explain/describe depression, but merely to predict whether it was likely to occur, and even an ill-theorized test can turn out empirically to have considerable predictive value.)

Research Paper 2: Dingwall and Fox (1986)

The second paper we review in this chapter is a comparison of health visitors and social workers, by Robert Dingwall and Susan Fox. This is clearly not an experiment: it is not possible to assign people randomly to be health visitors or social workers. However, the difference between the two groups is explored *as if* this were an experimental manipulation, to investigate their similarities and differences of attitude to cases of violence and neglect towards children.

Exercise 17

You may now like to read the paper – Robert Dingwall and Susan Fox (1986). 'Health visitors' and social workers' perceptions of child care problems', in A. While (ed.) *Research in Preventive Community Nursing Care*, published by Wiley. It is also reprinted in Abbott and Sapsford (1992).

The overall question behind the Dingwall and Fox research is what qualifications are needed to be an effective health visitor, and the perennial debate about whether health visiting more resembles nursing or social work:

> Need health visitors be nurses? . . . In part, of course, this question is too vague for any firm answer to be given. It all depends on what we want health visitors to do and how we propose to train them. A more sensible question, however, might be to ask what difference a nursing background makes to health visitors . . . there are significant areas of overlap between the work of health visitors and of other health and welfare occupations. By comparing their approaches to these areas we may get some indication of the extent to which a nursing background does influence health visiting practice.
>
> (Dingwall and Fox 1986: p. 179)

The area of overlap on which they choose to focus is the perception of child care problems.

The study is explicitly a small-scale one, focusing on potentially unrepresentative samples of 20 social workers and 20 health visitors, all working in the same prosperous small town in the South of England. The numbers, and the single geographical location, mean that the samples may not be taken as representative of either profession as a whole. Comparison is further complicated by the fact that the two samples were drawn in different ways: the health visitors were selected by an Assistant Director as a representative cross-section of her staff, while the social workers were volunteers. The authors correctly note, therefore, that:

> It is not claimed that this study is representative of national experience, but we do hope to establish the value of the approach and to show that the results are sufficiently interesting to justify further investigation.
>
> (pp. 179–80)

The research technique used is the rating of vignettes – brief descriptions of cases or circumstances. Twenty vignettes were selected from a larger set designed by Giovannoni and Becerra (1979) and tried out in North American research. (Examples: Vignette 1 was 'On one occasion the parent and child engaged in mutual masturbation'; Vignette 4 was 'The parents usually punish their child by spanking him with a leather strap, leaving red marks on his skin'; Vignette 7 was 'The parents feed only milk to their child. The child has an iron deficiency'; Vignette 13 was 'on one occasion the parents left their child alone all night'). Vignettes were presented to each subject in random order, and subjects were asked to rate the seriousness of their implications for a 4-year-old child on a 9-point scale.

Of the results, Dingwall and Fox report that:

> The striking features of these data is the lack of differences between health visitors' and social workers' perceptions of potential child care problems. Although there were certain background differences these did not produce associated differences in the interpretation of the vignettes.
>
> (p. 187)

In terms of policy implications, they suggest that the difference in training between social workers and health visitors, often quoted as the major source of difficulty in their collaborative working on cases, may not be the barrier that it appears, because the attitudes of the two professions actually appear very similar, at least with respect to this one important area of common working. They suggest that institutional barriers and traditions may be a more important obstacle to collaboration.

On the original question, of whether health visitors need to be nurses, their conclusion is that:

> . . . it does lead us to ask exactly what a nursing background is conributing to health visiting. A full answer would obviously involve a much bigger study over a greater range of topics. Even so, these findings should give some cause for reflection on the necessity of nurse training for health visiting. This is not to say health visiting could or should be collapsed into social work: there are good arguments why these functions should be separated. It may, however, be the case that a much broader pool of people could become satisfactory health visitors than is currently possible. Alternatively, perhaps we should be asking whether the clinical element of health visiting should be enhanced, perhaps creating a community paediatric nurse practitioner, to make better use of the expensive prior training investment than is currently the case.
>
> (p. 188)

This paper is a good example of what we sometimes call *quasi-experimental* analysis – a comparison like an experiment in form, and following the same logic as an experiment, but not truly experimental because the independent variable (the one which is supposed to have a causal effect) is not under the control of the researcher. In this case the dependent variable is identified as 'having a nursing background and training'. What we actually compare, however, is a group of health visitors and a group of social workers, and there are undoubtedly many other differences between them. If differences in outcome *had* been found, the researchers would have needed to examine each of these possible differences, to show that it was not the factor responsible for the difference in outcome. Some of them would have been very difficult to disentangle. How, for example, do we distinguish 'having or not having a nursing background' from other aspects of the two jobs? (Perhaps by finding groups of nurses with social work training, and/or social workers who originally trained as nurses?)

One more point to note is that, as in so many experiments and quasi-experiments, the outcome measure is more trivial, more artificial, less 'real and earnest', than the real thing for which it is taken as proxy. The 'vignettes' illustrate features of real cases, but they lack the detail, complexity and inevitable degree of moral dilemma inherent in the real case. Furthermore, 'ratings of seriousness' are not something which form a normal part of the jobs of either social workers or health visitors; they decide whether or not to intervene, and asking for a 'rating' which is not tied to action is a somewhat artificial request. Even to the extent that the vignettes did simulate real cases, they would still not be real cases; we can never be sure that what is done in response to a research task is what would be done in the real situation. Finally, it might be relevant to suggest that social workers and health visitors may have been demonstrating not so much a *professional* consensus as a *cultural* one; that is, it is possible that a sample of non-professionals would have rated the cases very similarly.

(You will find, incidentally, that what this kind of research is *called* varies according to the discipline from which the research emanates. In social research, studies which involve a controlled manipulation by the researcher are called 'experiments', while studies which depend on comparing naturally occurring cases are called 'quasi-experiments' or looked on as a kind of 'survey'. In medical and health research the former is often called a 'controlled trial' if it involves the testing of a drug or procedure, while studies comparing, for instance, otherwise similar people who do or do not have a given disease are referred to as 'case-control studies'.)

Summary: points for evaluation

1 Controlled trials, experiments and studies which are like experiments stand or fall by two factors:
   (a) clear definition and measurement of a dependent variable (the thing to be influenced) and one or more independent variables [the thing(s) doing the influencing];
   (b) ruling out all other possible explanations of any obtained changes in the dependent variable.
2 In quasi-experimental analysis ('case-control studies') both of these are likely to be problematic, but the researchers should do their best to convince us that other plausible explanations are ruled out.
3 The major way in which change is demonstrated, and a large class of other explanations for it ruled out, is by comparison between groups which differ on the independent variable – often a contrast between an 'experimental' group which receives some treatment and a 'control' group from whom it is withheld. The logic of the argument will work only to the extent that these groups are comparable.
4 In some studies a 'same subjects' design will be used, with the same person

participating, sequentially, in the 'experimental' and the 'control' condition. In this case, however, it is important to rule out explanations of observed changes in terms of changes in the people concerned – learning, fatigue, etc.

5 However perfect the design, experimental research very often suffers from a tendency to trivialize or 'artificialize' the real situation which it is seeking to simulate. This should be looked out for in evaluating such studies.

Exercise 18

Now re-read the two papers in the light of our comments.

Further reading

Women and psychiatry

Brown, George and Harris, Tirril (1978). *Social Origins of Depression: A Study of Psychiatric Disorder in Women*. London: Routledge and Kegan Paul.
Busfield, Joan (1991). *Women and Mental Health*. London: Macmillan.
Fulani, Leonara (ed.) (1988). *The Politics of Race and Gender in Therapy*. New York: Haworth Press.
Nairn, K. and Smith, G. (1984). *Dealing with Depression*. London: Women's Press.
Orr, Jean (ed.) (1987). *Women's Health in the Community*. Chichester: Wiley.
Penfold, Susan and Walker, Gillian (1984). *Women and the Psychiatric Paradox*. Milton Keynes: Open University Press.

Health visiting

Abbott, Pamela and Sapsford, Roger (1991). 'Health visiting: policing the family?', in Pamela Abbott and Claire Wallace (eds) *A Sociology of the Caring Professions*. Basingstoke: Falmer.
Clark, June (1981). *What do Health Visitors do?* London: Royal College of Nursing.
Dingwall, Robert (1977). *The Social Organisation of Health Visitor Training*. London: Croom Helm.
Drennan, Vari (1986). 'Talking to health visitors – perceptions of their work', in A. While (ed.) *Research in Preventive Community Nursing Care*. Chichester: Wiley.

6

Reading survey research

Surveys are about finding out what is there – asking questions or observing, and counting the answers. (This is far too simple a definition to encompass anything like the full range of survey research, as we shall quickly see, but it is a good starting point.) The 'ideal survey' is the 10-yearly Census of Population, when squads of interviewers (known as 'enumerators') receive standardized training, and then go out to find every household in the country and get the answers to a range of basic questions about the people living there. Most surveys are smaller in scale than this and cannot hope to reach every member of the population. What they do is to ask questions of a *sample* of the population and hope that this sample is representative – that what is true of the sample will be true of the population as a whole. The General Household Survey, for instance, is another large government survey, happening more frequently than the Census, which also asks for household composition and living standards, but of a randomly drawn sample of the population – quite a large sample, but only a small percentage of the people who *might* have been asked. If the sample is random and reasonably large, then we can have every confidence that it is reasonably representative.

Most surveys are smaller still – including the two at which we shall look in this chapter. They share two key issues with larger ones, however. The first is the question of representation: to the extent that a survey sets out to describe a population on the basis of a sample, it has to be able to demonstrate that the sample is likely to be representative of the population. The second is validity of measurement: the answers, which are ultimately recorded as numerical codes, have to have been produced by clear, appropriate questions, or 'measuring instruments' which really do measure what the researcher says they measure.

The first of the two surveys discussed below, by Abbott and Payne, may be seen as primarily descriptive, though looking to see if a particular worry is 'born out by the facts' rather than just 'describing in general'. However, many surveys are not just descriptive. They have a quasi-experimental element about them: they were set up to test some statement about differences between two or more groups, or the (causal) association of two variables. The Dingwall and Fox paper in the last chapter, which we described there as quasi-experimental, was a survey; *all* quasi-experimental analyses are also survey-based. In the same way the paper by George Choon and Suzanne Skevington below is a survey which explores quasi-experimentally the effects of gender on the gender stereotypes of male and female nurses.

Exercise 19

You may now like to read the first of the papers, Pamela Abbott and Geoff Payne (1992). 'Hospital visiting on two wards', in P. Abbott and R. Sapsford (eds) *Research into Practice: A Reader for Nurses and the Caring Professions*.

Research Paper 1: Abbott and Payne (1992)

This is a much abridged version of a report commissioned by the Plymouth Community Health Council in 1987. The Plymouth Health Authority had introduced open visiting at the Authority's hospitals in 1986, so that visitors would be able to come at any time between 2.00 pm and 8.00 pm. The nurses on the maternity unit at one major hospital approached the PCHC, suggesting that the new visiting arrangements were unsatisfactory. They argued that insufficient time was left for carrying out necessary nursing duties and for mothers to learn how to handle their new babies. It was also said that the mothers found the new arrangements tiring.

Questionnaires were prepared and administered to visitors and patients by a group of Polytechnic students, after a pilot run to try out the wording of questions. The original sampling design was that students were to attend the hospital at whatever time they could manage during visiting hours and approach every visitor and patient during a 2-week period. This proved impractical because of the rapid 'turn-round' on these kinds of ward, and 2 weeks was not long enough to collect a large enough sample for analysis, so the study was extended until data had been collected from 88 visitors and 90 patients. (Visitors were approached when they arrived and asked if they would be prepared to answer a few questions, then or later; patients were interviewed in their beds. The patients to be interviewed were selected in advance by nursing staff, to avoid those who were seen as too ill and to give those who did not want to participate a chance to refuse without embarrassment.) As a comparison, the researchers selected the gynaecological wards to set against the maternity wards. There had been no specific complaint from these, but they contained similar kinds of patient and were likely to be beset with some of the same problems. After the visitor and patient data had been collected, a self-completion questionnaire (with a reply-paid envelope) was sent to all the nurses and auxiliaries working on both wards.

Of the visitors who were interviewed, more than three-quarters were visiting the maternity wards. About half were male. Nearly 90 per cent were coming to see a close relative, and all but one of the remainder described the person being visited as a 'close' friend, not just a neighbour or acquaintance. Half the visitors came alone, and the rest accompanied by, mostly, one or two other people – for the most part other family members. No group of visitors included more than two children, and only 17 children in total accompanied adult visitors onto the wards. Visitors did not feel that either they or the visitors of other patients constituted too large a number or disrupted the ward, and there was little evidence that children or excessive numbers of visitors were perceived by other visitors as causing a nuisance.

The same was true, broadly, of patients. Most of those interviewed were visited regularly, generally by husbands or mothers. Forty per cent were visited by their own children, sometimes on a regular basis, but few were visited by children other than their own. Most of the patients thought that neither they nor others had too many visitors on the whole (though a few thought it might happen very occasionally), and few mentioned children as a particular problem (though some did find them noisy and unruly). There were no significant differences between the two types of ward.

Questionnaires were sent to all nurses, of whatever rank, on the two sets of wards, but only about a third were returned (rather more, in percentage terms, from the maternity wards than the gynaecological wards, which may reflect the greater concern in the former). The majority of those who filled in a questionnaire were registered nurses or midwives – and none of the sisters did so.

The majority on both kinds of ward felt that the existing visiting rules were satisfactory, but some expressed concern about the constant flow of visitors, with half a dozen or so round a bed at one time, giving neither the visited patients nor others on the ward any period of respite. Most of the nurses on either kind of ward could remember times when there were too many visitors in the ward, and when particular patients had too many visitors, and a substantial subset remembered occasions when there were too many children on the ward, creating a nuisance.

> . . . the children are often allowed to run up and down the corridors unchecked by their parents and so disturb other patients. [They] may also be prone to accident if not watched by their parents, as staff do not have time to watch that they do not get up to mischief or fall over etc.
> (Midwife, quoted in Abbott and Payne 1992)

Many of the maternity nurses could recall recent occasions when they felt visitors had stayed too long. About half had received complaints from patients – some about over-restrictive application of the rules, but more than half about their own or another patient's visitors. All but one of the maternity nurses had needed to ask visitors to comply with the rules – mostly excessive numbers or calling or staying outside the regular hours – and many had had occasion to speak to them about their behaviour on the ward.

Nurses were divided on how they thought the patients felt about the existing system – some thinking they liked it, some thinking that they would prefer greater freedoms, some that they would prefer more restriction (e.g. a break between afternoon and evening visiting). In terms of their own preference, most thought that permitted numbers should be increased, and all allowed that it was important that the patient's own children be allowed to visit (but most were more doubtful about other people's children). However, there was a sizeable minority, particularly on the maternity wards, who thought that the present system was not in the patients' best interests and/or interfered with nursing duties on the ward.

The authors recommended:

1 that the principle of open visiting would not be much compromised if time were found for a small meal-break for maternity unit patients;
2 that the rules could be slightly modified to allow more visitors and to allow for partners' needs to visit at varying times;
3 that the 'briefing' for partners and patients could be improved;
4 that brief formal training might be required, to give nurses insight into visiting as a legitimate part of the professional activity of the hospital and to improve their interpersonal skills so that they can handle 'difficult' visitors with more assurance.

Exercise 20

The second paper in this chapter, which you may want to read now, is George Choon and Suzanne Skevington (1984). 'How do women and men in nursing perceive each other?', in Suzanne Skevington (ed.) *Understanding Nurses*, published by Wiley: Chichester. A slightly shortened version is reprinted in P. Abbott and R. Sapsford (eds) (1992) Research into Practice: A Reader for Nurses and the Caring Professions.

Research Paper 2: Choon and Skevington (1984)

The theoretical base for this paper is the concept of sex stereotyping: the tendency of individual men and women to hold a shared, culturally determined picture of their own and the other gender. A number of studies are cited which show that within any given culture there tends to be a high degree of consensus about the nature of differences between the two sexes. Men are seen overall as more powerful – adventurous, realistic, independent, rational, aggressive – and women as more social or conciliatory – affectionate, appreciative, gentle, charming, weak, etc. Sex-linked characteristics are attributed to certain occupations, and among the occupations linked in the popular mind with 'being female' is that of the nurse. On the other hand, men also enter the nursing profession. So the research question is what nurses think of their own characteristics and those of opposite-sex nurses, and what they think the opposite gender, in its turn, thinks of them.

The target population was psychiatric nurses. The authors note that this may in some ways be untypical, because psychiatric nursing is not seen as a particularly female profession – men have been employed in it in substantial numbers for a very long time. On the other hand, it is a branch of nursing that *does* contain a substantial minority of men, so that any stereotypes that are formed by women stand a reasonable chance of being modified by real experi-ence of working with male counterparts, and the stereotypes formed by men should not be contaminated by the fact of being a very small minority in an essentially gendered branch of the profession. The research tool was the 'semantic differential', a series of adjective pairs which the subject applies to the object of categorization, scoring them as nearer to one pole or the other, or somewhere in the middle, on a 7-point scale.

> Twenty-one scales of this type were given to 99 psychiatric nurses (28 men and 71 women), and were used to find out what nurses thought about their own sex group and the other sex group, as well as what they thought the other group thought about them.
>
> (Choon and Skevington 1984: 106)

The results were that there was some tendency for each sex to stereotype its own members in the expected direction, but with some significant differences from expectation: women, for example, rated women as active and intel-ligent, while men rated men as co-operative, expressing anger verbally and cautious. When rating the other sex, however, something akin to the tradi-tional stereotypes emerged. The 'metaperspective' results – where subjects were asked to rate how the other gender would see theirs – were even more extremely sex-stereotyped. What was very noticeable was that the two genders agreed, roughly, on the characteristics of nurses in general, but these agreed characteristics were largely 'feminine', for male nurses as well as female ones.

The overall conclusion of the study is that:

> The present findings indicate that in terms of self-perceptions, percep-tions of the opposite sex, and beliefs of opposite-sex perceptions, there is a consistent and highly significant difference between male and female nurses, which might be attributable to sex-role stereotyping. Generally, the professional qualities popularly stereotyped as feminine . . . are highly rated by both female and male nurses in their self-perceptions. However, female nurses do not perceive male nurses to possess these qualities, and the perpetuation of such sex-role stereotypes in selection, training and professional practice may be damaging in preventing men from entering the profession.
>
> (p. 109)

However, this charge is qualified by recourse to existing structural factors:

> . . . it seems clear from the statistics that [men] are given highly preferen-tial treatment once trained, in a way that must make the talented woman

in nursing feel resentful and threatened, and even more determined to maintain nursing as women's work.

(p. 109)

Discussion

Three points are worth considering about these papers and all others of their kind, points which bear directly on our evaluation of published research. The first is the question of *measurement*. As we noted earlier, clear measurement of the quantities which are to be counted is quite essential for this kind of research. The Abbott and Payne paper comes off quite well on this criterion, on the face of it. The questions which were asked were obviously quite clear and 'factual' – times of day, numbers of visitors, numbers of children. One relies, of course, on the memory of the informant, but many of the questions were about this or immediately previous days' events, so memory should be trustworthy. The longer-term questions, about events which have happened in the past, are more suspect in this respect. Memory for the past is prone to inflation or diminution, depending on what point the informant thinks the survey is trying to prove. In survey research, no less than in less structured styles, the informant makes sense of the situation and tailors his or her replies to the sense that has been made.

A more general point may be made about 'measurement of the past' by survey means. The Abbott and Payne survey, like many others, is a *retrospective* one – it draws a sample now and asks them about what has happened over time. A better design, avoiding many of the problems of memory and mental reconstruction, would be a *prospective* survey or *cohort study*. In this design the researchers pick a sample at the beginning of a time period and follow them through to see what happens to them. For example, one of the best of the 'juvenile delinquency' studies did not take a sample of present criminals and explore their past, but took a random sample of all children of a certain age in a certain area and followed them forward to see who became delinquent and in what circumstances (West 1969; Knight and West 1975; West and Farrington 1975). The two drawbacks to prospective studies, however are:

1 they are costly – they take a long time, and a large sample is needed to allow for 'attrition' (loss of cases over time, through death, losing contact or eventual withdrawal of co-operation);
2 it is not always possible to apply this method – it is not clear, for example, that a prospective study would have been any more accurate than Abbott and Payne's retrospective one, given that the 'factual' questions about the past are really aimed at measuring what the nurse (for example) feels now that she has experienced, rather than 'what really went on'.

The measurement of gender stereotypes in the Choon and Skevington paper is not obviously straightforward. The test itself is quite simple – asking people to rate men and women on a list of adjectives. The task is an artificial one, however; we seldom sit and think about men or women as a class, with the intent simply of seeing whether a given adjective or its opposite best fits them. To the extent that we do, it is in very particular circumstances – generally single-sex derogatory conversations about the other sex, often sparked off by a quarrel or slight experienced by one member of the group. Thus, there is no knowing whether what is produced is what really rules our lives. Given no more information about the person than that he or she is male or female, perhaps these stereotypes have substantial force. Knowing that he or she is a nurse, or a teacher, or an engineer, or an accountant, or married or single, or black or white, or young or old, perhaps other sets of stereotypes may become more important. Having worked with the given person for a period of time, perhaps we make our judgements on a different basis altogether. There is also no detail in the report about precisely how the task was explained to the respondent and the instrument administered, which could make a substantial difference to the results.

Even within the Abbott and Payne study, some of the questions should not be taken as simply factual – those on 'how you feel about . . .' some aspect of the situation. How do you feel about reading this book, at this precise moment? Are you satisfied? Fairly satisfied? Neither satisfied nor unsatisfied? Puzzled about how to answer the question, given that some aspects of the book may be quite useful, but others are clearly tedious or over-simple? Puzzled about how to answer the question before you have finished reading it and had time to think about it and perhaps use it in other contexts?

The second substantial question, for evaluation, is the question of *representation (sampling)*. In the Abbott and Payne paper a real effort is made to obtain a representative spread of patients and visitors, insofar as the problems of those visiting in a particular month are typical of visitors during the rest of the year. It might have been better, if it had been possible, to sample the times of day systematically, but otherwise the sampling design cannot be faulted, and although it was not carried out perfectly in practice, no harm seems to have resulted. Of the nurses the same cannot be said. All nurses were approached, but only about a third replied, and we cannot say that this third were typical of the others. Indeed, we know they were not typical; the more senior staff were under-represented. (This is a standard problem of postal or self-completion questionnaires; the typically low response rate can make the results very suspect.) To the extent that the nurses, patients and visitors were typical for that particular establishment, the authors have fulfilled their purpose, which was to answer a question about that specific establishment. One might want to generalize the findings more widely, to other hospitals in the same Authority or to hospitals in general. The extent to which one may do so will depend on the extent to which the hospital, and its staff and patients were typical of others, and the authors do not discuss this question.

In the other paper, by Choon and Skevington, discussion of sampling is seriously inadequate. All we are told is that the informants were psychiatric nurses, and how many there were. We do not know how or from where they were selected and are, therefore, quite unable to say how typical they are of their profession.

The third point is the quasi-experimental nature of one of these papers, which always rests ultimately on an appeal to causation, and in all but the pure experiment/controlled trial on a more or less dubious appeal. In the Choon and Skevington paper, for example, the differences in semantic differential ratings are attributed to the gender of the informants – gender 'causes' direction and type of stereotyping. This is a likely conclusion, but formally speaking all we can show from a study such as this is that gender is correlated with it. There could be some other factor which provided a better explanation, which in turn is associated with gender – in this case, perhaps, the very different professional socialization experiences of male and female nurses might be a candidate. Because it is not possible to isolate gender from any other differences between the two groups, it is not possible to assert without fear of contradiction that it is the gender difference which causes the difference in attitude. As we said in the last chapter, this is a general problem of interpretation with 'case-control' research and the quasi-experimental analysis of survey data.

Summary: points for evaluation

1 In any piece of survey research one important question is how well the things which are being counted have been defined – how good the measurement is. There are four sub-questions which might follow from this:
   (a) Looking logically at the argument of the paper, have the right things been measured? (Are the concepts correctly *operationalized*?)
   (b) Are the factual questions clear and unambiguous, and how likely is it that the respondents have answered them accurately?
   (c) Where what is being asked is being taken as a measure or indicator of something underlying, is it a valid indicator? In other words, what is the proof that it does measure what it is claimed to measure?
   (d) Looking at the interview or recording session as a social situation of which respondents have to make sense, how likely is it that the sense they make of the task will lead to them giving the information which the argument of the paper needs (as opposed, for instance, to something which is specific to the interview situation and is not likely to have any bearing on any other part of their lives)?
2 If the paper is in any way quasi-experimental – seeks to show that something is an *effect* of something else – there will always be the possibility of alternative explanations, perhaps in terms of factors not even considered in the paper.
   (a) If the researchers have tried to eliminate particular alternative explanations, how good are their arguments?
   (b) What other factors might they have overlooked which are plausible or at least possible as alternative explanations?
3 How typical is the sample of the population to which the results are to be generalized?
   (a) Was the sampling carried out in such a way that it is likely to be representative, or by a method which makes bias likely?

(b) Were certain parts of the population excluded from consideration, either deliberately or accidentally (e.g. by non-response to a self-completion questionnaire), and what difference might that make to the conclusions?

Exercise 21

Now re-read the two papers in the light of our comments.

Further reading

Gender stereotyping

Abbott, Pamela and Wallace, Claire (1990). *An Introduction to Sociology: Feminist Perspectives*. London: Routledge.

Burns, R.B. (1977). 'Male and female perceptions of their own and the other sex' *British Journal of Social and Clinical Psychology*, 16, 213–20.

Fransella, Fay and Frost, K. (1977). *On Being a Woman*. London: Tavistock.

Hollway, Wendy (1989). *Subjectivity and Method in Psychology: Gender, Meaning and Science*. London: Sage.

7

Reading secondary-source research

Using secondary sources

Like most methods courses and textbooks, we have talked so far as if all research were a matter of going out and collecting fresh data. In fact, the most commonly practised kind of research involves illustrating or supporting an argument by reference to data which have already been collected by someone else, generally for some other purpose. This is known as the secondary use of data, and we refer to the sources as 'secondary sources'. Most commonly when we use the term we mean published numerical data – 'statistics', in the original meaning of the term, meaning numerical information about something of interest in the population. Possible sources range widely, from the statistics contained in other people's published research, through various kinds of regular survey such as the General Household Survey or the Census, and statistics collected for governmental research reasons (e.g. the incidence of certain kinds of infectious diseases), to statistics which are purely a by-product of the administrative process (criminal convictions, admissions to hospital, birth and death statistics, etc.) These are very good sources of information in that they can usually offer a degree of 'coverage' which is beyond the resources of the individual researcher or research team. It would not be possible for you, for example, to count every baby born in the country each year, but the government counts them routinely. The use of secondary sources presents special problems, however, precisely because it *is* a secondary use; we are often trying to use statistics for purposes for which they were not originally intended. We have to be especially careful, therefore, that the ones we use are *reliable* (i.e. an accurate count of what we want to count, collected in a consistent way), and *valid* for the purposes for which we want to use them.

As a case of unreliable statistics, we might briefly consider the statistics on suicide available from the government publication *Statistics of Deaths Reported to Coroners*. This gives a count of the number of cases where a coroner has determined (with or without the aid of a jury) that the cause of an unexplained death shall be recorded as suicide, and that is *precisely* what they count – not the 'real' incidence of suicide, whatever that may be.

1 Not all suicide cases, almost certainly, are reported to coroners in the first place. If the deceased was under the care of a doctor and the doctor certifies the death as being from natural causes, and no other person reports the death as suspicious to the coroner or to the Registrar of Deaths, then the case will never come to the attention of a coroner at all and, therefore, cannot appear in the statistics.

2 The coroner (and probably the police) will investigate cases of suspicious death before the inquest, and they may find sufficient evidence to justify a suicide verdict.

3 When all the evidence is in, the decision as to whether the case is a suicide, an accident or some form of homicide is a subjective one on the part of the coroner (or the jury, if one has been called), and therefore liable to be affected by the personal values of those taking it. This invalidates any sort of class or gender comparison even within one country, because it is all too likely that suicide will seem a more plausible explanation for one class than another, or one gender than another, on a systematic, culturally determined basis. It certainly invalidates comparisons *between* countries given, for example, the different social consequences of suicide in catholic and protestant countries.

4 At a more fundamental level, it is not possible even in principle to have an accurate count of suicides. We cannot ask the suicide whether he or she really meant to die. If we give any credence whatsoever to the concept of suicide attempts as cries for help, and allow that some attempts which if they had failed would be seen as 'not serious attempts' might accidentally succeed in killing the person concerned, then we cannot ever know whether the person in question died by deliberate self-slaughter.

5 Even if it had been possible to ask, or if an explanatory note has been left, we still cannot be quite sure, because one cannot be quite sure (given any idea of unconscious motivation) that even the victims themselves are in a position fully to explain their actions.

By contrast, the Census is a reliable source of information about the population. There are still some areas in which it may fall down. When counting households, for instance, it relies on its enumerators (data-collectors) to apply a definition of 'household' consistently, and despite subsequent checking we can never be quite certain that this has been done in the case of non-standard households. The count of the homeless is frankly suspect, being carried out by police officers going round the likely haunts of those who 'sleep rough' and trying to get what information they can. In the last instance, moreover, the accuracy of what is put on the form depends on the honesty and understanding of the individual informants. By and large, however, we would be prepared to accept the Census as one of the most reliable of data-sources.

The paper which we shall be considering in this chapter uses Census data to assess the material deprivation of small areas (wards) within the Plymouth

Health District. It then compares material deprivation with health status. Unfortunately, very few health statistics are collected and published on a routine basis. The major 'medical' statistics are the records of births and of deaths published in OPCS Monitors and other volumes (see Further Reading, at the end of this chapter). The authors have used death statistics, which may be trusted as reliable: all deaths must by law be notified to the authorities, and the official procedures have to be gone through before a body can legally be buried or cremated. (Cause of death, though also notified, is not reliable: there is too much variation in diagnostic practice.) Both these and Census data are available on request for quite small geographical areas, the 'wards', which permits fairly small-scale mapping.

There are still two preliminary concepts we need to look at first, before we go on to look at the research paper, because they are both used extensively in it. The first is the question of *standardization* or *normalization*, and techniques for doing it. If you have two sets of figures which are in some way unlike each other, you *standardize* when you do some simple (or sometimes not so simple!) arithmetic on them to make them easier to compare with each other. The simplest form of standardization is the familiar operation of expressing figures as percentages. If for example you were given the figures on the left of Table 7.1, which group of boys would you say was the greediest? Those in the first column ate more cakes, but there were also more of them. By percentaging, we eliminate (*control for*) the difference in number of boys, so that we can see clearly that it is Group B which ate proportionately more of their cakes – the figures on the right of the table. Then, in the final line of the table, another form of standardization is demonstrated – reducing the figures to a common base of cakes *per boy*, again showing that Group B were the greedier. Putting it another way, Group B's boys eat more cakes each, on average, than we would expect if we took Group A as typical.

One of the more impressive terms in the research paper we shall be considering is the *Standardised Mortality Ratio* (SMR). The SMR, as its name suggests, is a form of standardization, and it is similar in essence to the notion of 'cakes per boy' in Table 7.1. Eastbourne has a much higher death rate than the country as a whole – per thousand of population, more people die there in the

Table 7.1 Two illustrations of standardization. The boys in two groups were each given 10 cakes and told to save as many as they could, but to eat if they were very hungry

	Actual numbers		Percentages	
	Group		Group	
	A	B	A	B
No. of boys in group	5	2		
Number of cakes available	50	20		
Cakes eaten	15	8	30%	40%
Cakes eaten per boy	3	4		

course of a year than we would expect from looking at the death-rate for the population as a whole. On the other hand, it also has a larger than average population of pensionable age, so on the whole you would expect there to be more deaths. It is also well known that women are hardier than men at all stages of the life-cycle – less likely to die by any given age, and more likely to 'make old bones'. So if we wanted to look at how different Eastbourne's medical services are, using death-rates as a basis of comparison, it would hardly be fair to Eastbourne just to take crude death rate as our measure. What we do is to say arbitrarily that the SMR for the population as a whole is 100. Then we look at the area we want to analyse (Eastbourne) and see how its population compares with the country as a whole in terms of age and sex. For each age-band in each sex we work out a separate *age-and gender-specific death rate* for the population as a whole – what proportion of men aged 30–39 died in the population as a whole, for instance, what proportion of women aged 30–39, and so on. Then we apply these specific death-rates to the numbers in the population of Eastbourne to find out how many deaths we would expect if the age and gender structure of Eastbourne were the same as that of the whole population. We can then compare this 'expected figure' with the number who actually died, dividing the one by the other and then multiplying by 100. If the result is less than 100, then Eastbourne has fewer deaths than might have been expected. If it is larger than expected, then it has more deaths than might be expected. We can even say how much less or more: an SMR of 80 would mean that Eastbourne had only 80 per cent of the deaths we would expect if it were similar to the rest of the country in terms of age and sex balance; an SMR of 120 would mean it had 20 per cent more deaths than expected. (Eastbourne actually has a relatively low SMR: its hospital and community practitioners have considerable competence in geriatric medicine.) So the calculation of SMR may be difficult, but the basic idea is a simple one: do we have more or less deaths than we would expect after *controlling for* the effects of age and sex.

Normalization, a concept much used in the paper, involves some even more complicated arithmetic in practice, but again the basic idea is very simple and very similar to the above. When we want to compare two sets of figures which are expressed in different units or categories there are obvious problems. How do we compare overcrowding – expressed as the number of people in the average household divided by the number of rooms in the house – with the incidence of death, or low birth-weight babies, in the same area. The answer is that we do something rather similar to calculating an SMR. We take the *mean* (the average) of each variable for the overall area (in this case the Plymouth Health District), and call that zero. Then for each variable, from our list of the differing values for each ward, we calculate a quantity called a *standard deviation*, such that about two-thirds of the wards come out as within plus or minus one standard deviation of the mean – they are on the mean, or lower, or higher, but not more than one of these units lower or higher. We can then compare how *extreme* a ward is on each variable, compared with the Plymouth District as a whole, without worrying about the original units of measurement. If death-rate is associated with overcrowding, then if a ward is extreme in terms of death-rate we would expect it to be equally extreme in terms of overcrowding, and in the same direction away from the mean. If there is no association between the two, then overcrowding does not predict death-rate. (Using these *standard deviation* units, we count an area as extreme if it has a value of more than about 2, and as very extreme if it has a value of more than about 2.6.)

The second preliminary concept we need to explore is the idea of *correlation*. As we said above, two variables are said to be *associated* or *correlated* if there is a relationship between them such that extreme values on one predict extreme values on the other and a middling value on one predicts a middling value on the other. So height and weight are correlated: all things being equal, taller people weigh more. This is called *positive correlation*, with high values on one variable predicting high values on the other. *Negative correlation* occurs where high values on one variable predict low values on another: an example might be fitness and blood pressure – all things being equal, the less fit you are, the higher your blood pressure. *Perfect* correlation (positive or negative), is said to occur when the values of one variable exactly predict the values of the other – distance covered in a given time is perfectly correlated with speed of running (by definition). Perfect correlation is seldom found in social research, however. When we say that height and weight are correlated, we do not mean that all tall people are heavier than all people shorter than them, but that on the whole the heaviest people will be among the tallest.

The *correlation coefficient* is a mathematical way of expressing the degree to which two variables are correlated – tedious to calculate, but quite easy to understand. A coefficient of correlation carries the value of $+1.0$ if there is perfect positive correlation between the two variables, -1.0 if there is perfect negative correlation, and zero if there is no correlation at all. The values in between express the degree and direction of correlation, so $+0.7$ is a reasonably high degree of positive correlation, and -0.2 a reasonably low degree of negative correlation. For those who like playing with their calculators, if you square the correlation coefficient (i.e. multiply it by itself) and multiply the answer by 100, you get *percentage of variance explained*. (The 'variance' is the amount the figures differ among each other.) A perfect correlation of 1.0 or -1.0 explains 100 per cent of the variance. A correlation coefficient of zero explains none. The correlation of 0.7 above explains 49 per cent of the variance, and the one of 0.2 only 4 per cent.

The paper we are going on to examine is full of correlation coefficients. Sometimes these are combined into *multiple correlation coefficients*, which are quite simply the correlation of more than one variable with a dependent variable, all at the same time. So weight might be correlated with height and, quite separately, gender might be correlated with height. The multiple correlation would be the simultaneous effects of gender and weight together on the prediction of height – the extent to which being a heavy woman as opposed to a heavy man predicts whether you are likely to be taller or shorter. The multiple correlation coefficients are calculated for the paper by a procedure called *stepwise multiple regression*, which adds the variables to the prediction one at a time, starting with the one that has the most effect and working down, so that one can see which are the most important predictors, and which of the variables have no effect on the prediction once the effect of the others is taken into account.

Exercise 22
You might now read Abbott *et al.* (1992). 'Health and material deprivation in the Plymouth Health District', in P. Abbott and R. Sapsford (eds) *Research into Practice: A Reader for Nurses and the Caring Professions*. Alternatively, you may wish to read the original report (of which this is a substantially abridged re-edition) edited by Pamela Abbott (1988) and published by Polytechnic South West (see Further Reading). In either case you should not spend too long at it or get too involved in the statistics. Read it for the main conclusions and an understanding of the main methods used to achieve them. Look at the detail of the methods only where it is comes easily to you or you need it to understand the conclusions or how they were reached.

Research Paper: Abbott *et al.* (1992)

Two national studies of health and health inequalities have had a very profound impact on discussions of health provision in this country. The first was the Black Report (Townsend and Davidson 1980), the report of a government-inspired enquiry into the causes of unequal health status, which strongly suggested that structural inequalities such as social class were far more strongly correlated with inequalities in health status than any attitudinal or life-style variables. The second, *The Health Divide* (Whitehead 1987), showed that the inequalities noted in the Black Report, and their structural basis, were the same or worse 10 years later.

An incidental conclusion of both reports has been that there are substantial geographical inequalities in health status. This conclusion has given rise to a number of 'mini-Black Reports' which look at geographical health inequalities in more detail within smaller areas and conclude that there can be quite marked differences even within quite small geographical districts. Studies have been carried out in Glasgow, Edinburgh, Sheffield, Bristol and London, among other places, and even (Marsh and Channing 1986) within a single general practice.

> Area of residence has long been associated with mortality and morbidity. In Britain there exists a health gradient from North to South, death rates being highest in the North and West and lowest in the South and East . . . There is also an intra-regional gradient, with inner-city areas having higher mortality rates than rural areas . . . there are also differences between wards in the inner city, the wards with high SMRs being located in the most deprived areas, with the outlying suburbs . . . having lower SMRs for preventable deaths . . .
>
> (Abbott *et al.* 1992)

This examination of the Plymouth Health District (PHD) should be seen as another example of this kind of study. Its particular interest is that the PHD, which stretches across large sections of south-west Devon and across the Tamar into Cornwall, contains one substantial city with marked class gradients between fairly clearly delineated sections, plus rural areas of varying degrees of remoteness and varying degrees of affluence, so that there is a full range of types of areas for comparison. The south-west as a whole shows good health in comparison with the rest of Britain, so the existence of pockets or larger areas where this trend is reversed would be of particular interest to health administrators.

Even in the Black Report, social class (i.e. occupational status) was not seen as a variable which directly caused mortality or ill health, but rather as an indicator of materially deprived styles and circumstances of life. It happened to be a conveniently available indicator, being routinely recorded for all households in the Census and most other large-scale surveys. In later studies, however, attention has increasingly turned to more directly relevant indicators of material deprivation. The Census does not record household income or even income of head of household, but there are several variables which it does record which can be useful in assessing material state – ownership of cars, refrigerators or other 'consumer durables', number of people as compared with number of rooms in households (i.e. overcrowding), whether houses are owned or rented, and if the latter then whether they are rented within the private sector or from a council or housing association, and so on. The Plymouth study followed Townsend and his colleagues (e.g. Townsend *et al.* 1985, 1986a) in using a mix of 'indicators of deprivation'.

1 *Unemployment* – percentage of potentially employed residents aged 19–59 or 64 (according to gender) who were, in fact, unemployed.
2 *Car ownership* – the percentage of private households without the use of a car [found by Townsend *et al.* (1986b) to be a quite good indicator of level of income in urban areas].
3 *Home ownership* – the percentage of private households which were not owner occupied.
4 *Overcrowding* – the percentage of private households with more than one person per room.

All of these variables were derived from the 1981 Census small area data. The different items correlate quite reasonably with each other – at around 0.5, which means they share about a quarter of each other's variance. Given that some of the remaining variance is necessarily contributed by measurement error and the crudity of the indicators, and that they *are* only indicators and not direct measures, this suggests that there is, indeed, one underlying variable, giving support to the concept of material deprivation with which the authors started.

Social class itself was not included, despite its frequent use in previous studies:

In previous research social class has been used as a proxy indicator of disadvantage . . . there are problems, however, in using household social class . . . wide variation in salaries/wages between occupations within the same social class means that [it] is not necessarily a good indicator of income differentials. There is also the fact that [it] is based on the occupation of the 'head of household' and does not take account of the occupations of other members of the household. The increased proportion of wives in paid employment and making an economic contribution to the household means that households in the same social class can have widely differing levels of income.

(Abbott *et al.* 1992)

The indicators of health status which have been used in this paper are:

1 *Mortality* – SMRs for those of both sexes for people aged 1–65, averaged over a 5-year period. The deaths of the very young are dealt with by a separate indicator. The exclusion of the elderly is intended to focus the measure on 'avoidable death' and exclude the age-ranges where the death-rate climbs in any case; otherwise, the deaths of pensioners might swamp the analysis. The averaging over 5 years is to overcome chance fluctuations in areas where numbers are small.
2 *Disablement* – the proportion of all residents aged 16 or over living in private households who classed themselves as permanently sick or disabled.
3 *Infant mortality* – the rate of death of infants aged less than 1 year, per thousand live births, again averaged over a 5-year period.

The first and third come from mortality statistics obtained from *OPCS*. The second is from the Census and was the only health-related question which the 1981 Census asked.

Each of the sets of indicators was combined into a single variable, respectively 'material deprivation' and 'health status'. The method adopted was to 'normalize' each set of figures – to express them as having a mean of zero and units which are standard deviations – so that they are comparable as measures of extremity (see above), and to add the values so obtained. The resultant figures were then re-normalized so that the composite measures each had a mean of zero, and 1 unit of the new measure equalled 1 standard deviation of the old measure. This enables one to see just *how* extreme some wards are on one or the other measure, or both.

Looking at the composite variables separately, very substantial differences were found among the wards of the PHD. No ward scored exceptionally low on material deprivation, though some of the eastern suburbs (old small towns and villages now incorporated in the city) and one or two of the rural areas of south-west Devon close to the main trunk road came out as substantially more affluent than the average. On the other hand, there were five wards which showed a very high material deprivation score, and one which had an exceptionally high score. These were all urban wards, mostly those surrounding the dockyards. On the composite indicator of health status, again there were no extremely good scores, though several wards (mostly rural) showed themselves as enjoying considerably better health than the average, but four inner-city wards scored very badly on this variable.

The results show substantial association between material deprivation and health status. To a large extent the same wards came out as extreme on both measures – more so for the 'poor' wards than for the 'affluent' ones. Eight wards, all in the inner city, were in the top 20 per cent of scores on both material deprivation and health status – i.e. exhibited a degree of poverty and of poor health. Six wards were in the lowest 20 per cent on both measures. The two measures produce a correlation coefficient of 0.64, so material deprivation predicted about 40 per cent of the variance in health status. This is a very substantial proportion, given that we have only indicators rather than direct measures and that the indicators are crude.

One thing that emerged very clearly, and suggests a fruitful line for further research, is that health status was substantially more predictable in urban than in rural areas using these indicators. Looking at the correlation between material deprivation and health status separately for urban and rural wards, the authors found that the prediction for urban areas was much higher than for the area as a whole – 60 per cent of the variance was explained – but that the correlation for rural areas was very much lower and not statistically significant at all. It was noted that there was a much higher tendency for the separate indicators of deprivation to cluster together in urban wards than in rural ones, suggesting that not quite the same thing may be being measured. In urban wards, for example, it has been shown that access to a car is a quite good indicator of available financial resources. This may be much less true in rural wards – particularly the more remote ones – where, given the paucity of public transport, possession of or access to some sort of private transport may be an absolute prerequisite for being in work at all, however poorly paid that work.

> To sum up . . . it is possible to determine deprived areas (wards) in urban areas – areas where a high proportion of the population are deprived relative to the rest of the PHA. It is not possible to do this well for the rural wards using the same indicators . . . That the association between health status and material deprivation, as measured here, seems more tenuous for rural than for urban areas suggests to us that more research is required . . . no individual indicator of material deprivation was significantly associated with rural health status – despite the fact that all indicators are highly correlated. That deprivation and health status are not associated in rural areas seems unlikely. More likely is either that different measures of deprivation are needed . . . reflecting different lifestyles and different structural factors, or that the ward is an inappropriate level of aggregation for the study of rural health status.
>
> (Abbott *et al.* 1992)

Discussion

The problem with normalizing data, of course, is that it destroys the basis of comparison with other studies. When we speak above of wards being exceptionally deprived or having better or worse than average health status, the comparison takes the PHA as a baseline. We can say that a ward is better or worse than the PHA average, or exceptional in terms of the distribution of PHA wards, but we cannot directly compare the scores on the composite measures with those elicited for other areas by other researchers. What the researchers *have* done, however, is to compare the least and most deprived wards with figures for wards in London derived from Townsend *et al.* (1986b), using the individual deprivation indicators as the basis of comparison. The worst five wards in Plymouth were almost comparable with the worst five wards in the GLC (three of which were in Tower Hamlets). The percentage unemployed is entirely comparable, and the Plymouth wards were little better in terms of home ownership or availability of cars, although they were substantially better in terms of overcrowding. At the other extreme, however, the affluent Plymouth areas were not nearly as affluent as the affluent GLC areas (in Surrey, mostly). The Plymouth wards had a similar rating on overcrowding (virtually none), but scored substantially higher on percentage unemployed, percentage who were not home owners and percentage who did not have access to a car.

Studies of this kind rely on correlation to suggest causation, and this is a risky procedure, as we indicated in the previous chapter. Correlation is *necessary* for causation: if the supposed independent variable is not correlated with the dependent variable, then it cannot be a cause of it. Correlation is not *sufficient* for causation, however: two variables may be correlated without one being a cause of the other. A further problem is inherent in studies such as this whose basic unit of analysis is the geographical area rather than the person, because it does not follow that all those living in an area will share its characteristics. To treat the results as if this did follow is known as the *ecological fallacy*.

If an area shows a high level of deprivation, it does not necessarily follow that all the people in that area are deprived; wards are large enough areas that even the 'deprived' ones have pockets of wealth and gentrification, and even the 'non-deprived' ones have some areas of poverty and deprivation . . . Even in a relatively homogenous area there will be some well-off people living among the deprived or some poor people among the wealthy. Thus we cannot say absolutely that identifying a deprived area or an area of poor health is the same as identifying the people/households who are deprived or in poor health. Where health and deprivation correlate we cannot even say absolutely that it is the deprived people who have poor health, though this seems extremely likely. All we can assert with confidence is that if areas of high deprivation are also areas of poor health, then 'targeting' these areas in terms of resource provision should mean putting resources within the reach of a larger than average number of those who most need them.

(Abbott *et al.* 1992)

The authors also express reservations about the quality of their basic data:

There are . . . practical constraints on the use of the data derived from Census small area statistics which restrict their usefulness for rural wards. First, rural wards have small populations; and the small area statistics are derived from a ten per cent sample of the Census, not the full data-set. Thus they may sometimes be unrepresentative of the ward population as a whole. Secondly, ward boundaries are arbitrary and do not necessarily indicate discrete communities or homogeneous areas.

(Abbott *et al.* 1992)

Secondly, they express reservations about the use of mortality statistics as a major indicator of poor health; conditions which lead to death are a very specialized subset of the health problems with which people may be plagued.

The problem is that mortality figures may tell us that people live longer in the rural areas but they do not indicate whether rural people suffer more or less of those everyday illnesses that do not result in death or which the major part of the health services have to deal with.

(Fearn 1987, quoted in Abbott *et al.* 1992)

Thus, what we have here, as in many other similar studies, is an attempt to use less than ideal data to explore an important question. Overall the findings suggest very strongly that there is a strong association between material deprivation and health status, despite the crudity of some of the indicators. The results are definite enough to inform social policy – they point quite clearly to a direction in which money spent would not be wasted. As regards the academic study of causes of poor health, however, they must be taken as strongly suggestive rather than definitive. Apart from weaknesses in the data used in this study, the whole approach is quasi-experimental – it capitalizes on existing situations, and any number of variables which are not included in the study may be confounded with the nominated independent variables. While the association is so suggestive that it clearly calls for political action, in academic terms, we would like to see some indication of the *mechanism* by which one structural variable transforms itself into another before arguing that the case was proven.

Summary: points for evaluation

1 With secondary-source material, as with any other data, it is very important to understand just how the 'facts' have been collected and to be able to assess the reliability of the source – whether it works accurately and consistently in its data-collection.
2 With secondary sources even more than other forms of data the question of

validity arises – whether what has been collected quite corresponds to what the researcher wants to use the data for.

3 With secondary-sources data as with other survey-based sources, we should note that the argument which is put forward tends to be based on correlational or quasi-experiment logic. Arguments of this kind can be very strongly suggestive, but they do not, strictly, establish causation beyond doubt.

4 However, it is quite possible for an argument of this form to be so strongly suggestive that it may be worth altering social policy and spending social resources on the basis of it. We should always ask ourselves what we can *do* on the basis of findings as well as what we can *conclude*.

Exercise 23

Now re-read the paper in the light of our comments.

Further reading

Vital statistics

A basic source of statistics on birth, death, disease, marriage etc. is the OPCS *Monitor* series, of which specific annual issues deal with specific topics:

DH2 Deaths, by cause
DH4 Deaths from accidents and violence
DH5 Infant and perinatal death statistics
MB2 Infectious diseases
FM1 Birth statistics
FM2 Marriage and divorce statistics

Birth and death statistics may also be found in the OPCS publications *Social Trends* and *Population Trends* (or, for Northern Ireland, *Health and Personal Social Services Statistics for Northern Ireland* and the *Annual Report of the Registrar General for Northern Ireland*). Statistics on illness may be found in *Health and Personal Social Services Statistics*.

Deprivation and health status

Abbott, Pamela (ed.) (1988). *Material Deprivation and Health Status in the Plymouth Health District*. Plymouth: Polytechnic South West, Department of Applied Social Science.

Jarman, Brian (1983). 'Identification of underprivileged areas' *British Medical Journal*, 286, 28 May, 1705–9.

Johnson, I.S. *et al.* (1987). *Health Care and Disease: A Profile of Sheffield*. Sheffield: Sheffield Health Authority.

Townsend, Peter, Davidson, Nick and Whitehead, Margaret (1990). *Inequalities in Health*. Harmondsworth: Penguin. (Contains both The Black Report and The Health Divide.)

☰ **Section 3** ☰

Doing research

8

Using secondary sources

Using libraries – review of 'literature'

Most research reports begin with a section (or sections) which outlines the area of research, explains why it is interesting and/or important, and probably summarizes what is known so far and what the research which is reported has to offer which is new or different. Readers need to know what you can take for granted and build on, and why you choose to look at the problem in the way that you do. For the construction of this section of a report you will have to use the resources of libraries. In fact, you would almost certainly want to do so at a much earlier stage of the research. Reading past research reports and descriptive papers, and more theoretical articles and books, is an important part of the process of refining the research problem and forming ideas about how to carry out the research.

From your point of view, libraries come in two kinds – public and academic. The libraries of universities, polytechnics, colleges and schools of nursing are the better stocked from the point of view of carrying out a search through the 'literature', and if you are a registered student you will have automatic rights to use them. If you are not, however, your access will be limited. Most will allow you reading rights – to look at books and journals on the premises – and some will allow you to borrow books. Many will charge for the privilege. You will have to ask the librarian what is allowed in the particular library which is convenient for you. Public libraries are more accessible, and the larger branches will have some of what you need, but you are unlikely to find that they carry a large stock of publications of the kind for which you are looking.

In both kinds of library you will find:

- Books, generally arranged according to a subject-based cataloguing system.
- Journals, newspapers and other 'periodicals'.
- The Catalogue, which lists what the library stocks, by author, title and often subject area.

- Abstracts (volumes which contain a complete year-by-year list of publications in a certain area, by author and title, with a brief summary of contents, and generally an index classified by subject-matter to help you locate useful works); for example, *Nursing Abstracts* lists and describes a wide range of research on nursing.
- Annual 'review journals' – for example, *Research in Nursing and Health*.
- Other 'bibliographic instruments' – e.g. lists of published works such as *British Books in Print*.
- There is a national 'borrowing network' based on the British Library, a copyright library which receives copies of everything published in this country and also acquires quite a range of works published abroad. Books can be borrowed, and photocopies of journal articles obtained, by what is called 'Inter-Library Loan', and you should talk to the librarian if you need this. Be warned, however, that it can often take quite a lot of time to obtain books or articles by this means, and that there may often be a quite substantial fee for the service unless you are a registered student.
- The library of the Royal College of Nursing, in London, has a very large collection of relevant publications. People doing research on health and nursing should contact them if their local facilities are meagre or their subject-area a very specialized one.

In general, the most useful resource of all in a library is the librarians, who are generally very willing to help the student or researcher.

There are four main 'tricks' for homing in on relevant books and articles reasonably quickly:

1 Identify the catalogue reference which most closely fits the subject-matter of your enquiry (asking the librarian's help if necessary) and just look along the shelves at this point to see what the library has. You will be interested in anything which is fairly recent and/or which obviously bears closely on the question which underlies your research.
2 Browse through the last couple of years' issues of relevant journals – ones which are obviously, by their title, relevant to your work, and ones which you have noticed crop up quite often in the reference lists of other papers and books which you have been reading. (Don't neglect the book reviews, nor publishers' advertisements for books about to be published.)
3 Starting from papers which you have read and found useful, look in the reference lists to identify other articles or books which may be relevant. If they are, when you read them, then look in their reference lists in turn for other works. Then look through current journals or Abstracts (see below) for the most recent work by the same authors.
4 Use the subject index of the major series of Abstracts in your field (ask the librarian if you're not sure) to identify further relevant references. This is the most comprehensive stratagem, but the riskiest in the short term, because you may put in a lot of work locating papers or books which turn

out not to be of immediate relevance. It is a relevant way to proceed if you are writing a book or thesis, or if you are stuck for any references whatsoever, but on the whole it is not a good way to start.

Exercise 24: Literature search

If you have access to a reasonably large library, try your hand at an embryonic literature search. Take one of the papers you read in Part 2 which interested you, and try to identify and locate further articles or books which bear on the same topic.

Finding statistics

A part of the 'literature review' of any research paper will generally comprise an attempt to set the object of study in its context – to say how many of the people concerned there are, what proportion of the population they form, and in general how big the problem is. For this we need the figures which are collected by governmental and other bodies, published and made available in libraries – annual reports of government departments, figures routinely presented to Parliament, regular governmental surveys of the population or the economy or the institutions for which government is responsible. We may also need such figures to show how typical or representative our research samples are of the population which they purport to represent. Indeed, as we saw in the last chapter, it is quite possible to conduct an entire research project on such 'secondary' data. Often it will be the case that using already available statistics is the best way of tackling a research problem; the figures generally give a breadth of coverage that would not be available to the individual researcher without the expenditure of very large amounts of money and time.

Very often the figures you need will be in one or other of the regular annual summary publications. *Social Trends* produces annual 'headline' figures from a wide range of statistical sources and gives an overall picture of the 'state of the nation'. Detailed figures on births, marriages, deaths, family formation and so on can be found in the monthly *Population Trends*, and more localized figures are available in *Regional Trends*. These often include articles analysing and commenting on trends. For the audience of this book, the annually published *Health and Personal Social Services Statistics* is also likely to be an important source.

For more detailed work and for statistics which are harder to find, the 'bible' of the secondary-source researcher is the *Guide to Official Statistics* published from time to time by CSO, the Central Statistical Office. This gives an annotated list of virtually all sets of published official statistics, and some statistics published by non-governmental bodies. Consulting the *CSO Guide* is a normal first step in any secondary-source research, unless you already know your sources very well.

Population and vital statistics

The major source of statistics on the population and its demographic characteristics is the Census, held every 10 years. (We have already looked at this briefly in the last chapter.) The Census asks every household questions about who is present on Census night, who is usually present, their age, marital status, country of birth, employment, means of transport to work, educational qualifications, where they used to live, the details and amenities of their living accommodation, etc. It is the best source for reliable and authoritative information on the population of a given area and their housing. Results are presented on a regional basis and by county, as well as in national terms (for some of the analyses), and statistics of smaller areas are available on request, in tabular form or in a form amenable to computer analysis. (Some of the more complex analyses are carried out not on the full returns, but on a sample of them.) A limited range of statistics are also available for Local Authority Areas, urban areas, political constituencies, and even wards and parishes.

Happening every 10 years, the Census is inevitably out of date for large parts of a decade. More recent information (though generally based on samples rather than the whole population) may be obtained from the monthly OPCS publication *Population Trends*, from *Regional Trends* if geographically more specific information is required and from the annual *Social Trends* if all that is required is a broad overview. The other main source of descriptive population statistics, also carried out by OPCS, is the *General Household Survey*, a sample survey of a panel of households which asks some of the questions covered in the Census, but also more detailed ones on household amenities and income. A report of the survey is published annually.

There is a strict legal requirement for births and deaths to be reported, so these are among the most reliable of the published statistics. *Population Trends* gives numbers of births and deaths by age and gender, noting also numbers of stillbirths and of illegitimate births, and broad summary figures are also given in the annual *Social Trends*. More detailed figures are given in various of the OPCS *Monitors*; you should consult the CSO *Guide* for a list of these. Figures are often given as rates per thousand or ten thousand of the population (or of women of child-bearing age, in the case of births), a more useful way of representing them than simple raw numbers. Death-rates may be further adjusted to take account of the age and sex structure of the population under examination – the *standardized mortality ratio* discussed in the previous chapter, set at 100 if the group or region's adjusted death-rate is identical to the national average. Some statistics for Scotland and Northern Ireland will be found in *Population Trends*, but the major sources here are the *Annual Report of the Registrar General, Scotland* and *Annual Report of the Registrar General (Northern Ireland)*.

Health and the National Health Service

There are no systematic statistics on the health or disease of the population, but only records of particular illnesses or causes of death. A variety of death figures are available – childhood deaths at various stages around and before birth, causes of death as recorded on death certificates, deaths from accident or violence, occupational mortality, etc. These are reported in *OPCS Monitors* and in a variety of other publications (see the list at the end of the previous chapter and the *CSO Guide* for more detailed and up-to-date information). Certain infectious diseases have to be reported, and figures for these are given in *Health and Personal Social Services Statistics for England* (or comparable publications for the other countries of Great Britain – see the *CSO Guide*), as are reported cases of sexually transmitted diseases, registered cases of cancer and notifications of congenital malformation. This source also gives numbers of reported pregnancies and numbers of abortions carried out. The *General Household Survey* asks questions on smoking in even-numbered years and publishes the results, and the 1980 and 1982 volumes include data on drinking (which is also covered in summary form in *Social Trends*). Again there are more detailed sources of information which offer a range of analyses, and you should consult the *CSO Guide* for a list of them.

Statistics on the working of the Health Service are somewhat more comprehensive. Numbers of personnel in the hospital, family practitioner committee and community health branches of the Service, and local authority social service, are given in *Health and Personal Social Services Statistics*, as are costs, sources of finance and charges to patients or clients, and a breakdown of hospital beds by location and department. This volume also gives figures on use of hospital treatments, and the age and gender of patients, numbers of general practitioners, the number and cost of prescriptions dispensed, numbers of dentists and incidence of dental treatment, numbers of ophthalmic practitioners and the use (and cost) of their services, the numbers and usage in the ambulance service, and numbers in the school health service and the number of pupils inspected. There are cognate publications for Scotland, Wales and Northern Ireland, and many more specialized sources dealing with particular aspects of the service – again, see the *CSO Guide*.

Social services statistics

The major source here is *Health and Personal Social Services Statistics for England* (and comparable sources for the other countries of the British Isles – see the *CSO Guide*). This gives details of personnel and all the services which have been provided – domicilliary services, residential services, children and young persons in local authority care, housing and homelessness, etc. It also gives numbers of adoptions of children. *Local Government Financial Statistics* gives financial data on the personal social services. Again there are more detailed sources, for which you should consult the *CSO Guide*.

Exercise 25: Exploring secondary data

If you have an adequate library available, why not spend a few hours seeing what you can get out of available statistics. Pick some limited area of enquiry, look for relevant figures in the overall summary volumes such as *Social Trends*, look in the *CSO Guide* to see what else might be available and follow it up.

Problems with published statistics

Published statistics are a very strong source of information – the only available one for making comparisons over extended periods of time, unless you have a very long time in which to conduct your research, and with a 'sample size' that you are very unlikely to be able to match. There are problems, however, connected with the ways in which they are assembled and the purposes for which they are collected, which mean they have to be treated with even more caution than other sources of information.

The first problem is the question of *reliability*: are the statistics collected in a consistent way, so that one year's figures are comparable with another's? There may be several stages in a statistic's 'history' at which an individual's discretion comes into play, and this could be exercised in different ways from year to year, from place to place and from person to person. There are also gross changes of law, practice and the state of knowledge to contend with. Diagnosis of disease or handicap, for example, depends on someone presenting himself or herself to a doctor, who then exercises medical judgement as to whether a diagnosable condition is present and, if so, what it is. There are advances of medical knowledge which will change particular diagnostic practice from time to time. It may also be influenced by more social factors. For example, now that there are incentives to doctors for screening of women for cervical cancer, cases will be diagnosed earlier and there will be a temporary rise in the statistics – fewer cases will wait for the diagnosis until the condition becomes acute. The government statistics on numbers of deaths are reliable, being taken from counts of death certificates. The statistics on cause of death are also taken from death certificates, however, and these are *not* reliable: they depend on the potentially fallible diagnosis of doctors, plus an additional level of 'clerical discretion', where more than one cause is recorded and a clerk will have to decide which to take as the primary one. All survey questions – even apparently simple ones such as 'How would you describe your ethic origin?' Or 'Have you ever been raped?' – have to be scrutinized to see whether fashions in avowal or differential pay-offs for answering one way or the other might change the pattern of answers over time, even if the underlying 'facts' had not changed. Information collected by some government department, often for quite different purposes, needs to be scrutinized even more carefully.

This leads into the question of *validity* – do the statistics measure what they purport to measure? Putting it another way, is what they measure what *you* want to consider in your research? Diagnostic statistics, for example, measure not the extent of a given disease, but the extent to which it has been diagnosed, and diagnosis is not an automatic process, but one involving human decision-making. The statistics are very likely to be correlated with the real extent of disease – to go up when it goes up and down when it goes down – but the relationship could be quite a loose one, and small changes are as likely as not to be the result of a change in reporting or recording practice. So we need to remember that what we are measuring is, in part, a social construction, not a 'fact', and that there is error in the figures.

Another aspect of the validity question concerns the way that we tend to use what is available, even if it does not quite match up to what we need. In the Abbott *et al.* paper discussed in the last chapter the authors had to use mortality and registered disablement as their health measures, because this was what was available, but they were well aware that these are very crude health indicators and take no account of the great amount of human suffering and misery caused by 'lesser' complaints. We might assess the efficiency of hospitals by their throughput of patients and/or the number of patients treated for a given cost, but this would take no account of the *quality* of treatment. It is very easy to distort the original research question in the interests of using available statistics, or even to miss the core of it altogether.

The moral is that we must always scrutinize the secondary statistics which we are considering with at least as much care as we would scrutinize methods of data-collection we intend to use ourselves first-hand. Are the figures likely to be consistently and reliably collected? Do they measure what they purport to measure? Do they measure what *we* want to measure? Will the use of them in any way distort or prejudice the analysis of the original question? If so, what other figures can we use to overcome this, or what research ought we to go on and do to supplement what we can learn from the figures?

'Qualitative' sources

We have talked so far as if all secondary analysis is carried out on published statistics. It is also possible, however, to do qualitative secondary analysis, looking at what people have written or what has been written about them. Studying social policy, for example, government reports and white papers can be a rich source of information, and for more detailed work one can go to the newspapers (*The Times* and *The Guardian* have an annual index which makes it relatively easy to track down the date of 'policy events') or to *Hansard*, the daily record of what is said in Parliament. Professional journals can also be very useful in this respect. One should remember that what is presented is what the policy-makers *say* – how they justify what they are doing – and the criticisms that have been made from a range of entrenched positions; such work is seldom to be taken as a purely factual source of information. In this, however, they differ little from any other qualitative source; it is always necessary to remember that people give *accounts* of their lives and actions, not straight factual reports.

With this same qualification, people's own personal accounts can also help to 'flesh out' figures or can be used as a source in their own right:

autobiographies, published collections of letters, diaries, even novels can help to give some feel for what a situation or condition is like 'from the inside' in circumstances where interviewing is not possible. One may also go to reports of ethnographic research for summarized accounts of other people's interviewing. Thus, the literature review can also be a form of data-collection.

Exercise 26: Exploring qualitative sources

Taking the topic which you explored in Exercise 25, spend a few hours in a large library looking for anything qualitative which bears on it – diaries, letters, autobiographies, ethnographic research reports, official pronouncements. (In other words, get started on a literature review.) See what these add to the quantitative material you have developed.

Further Reading

Hindess, Barry (1973). *The Use of Official Statistics in Sociology*. London: Macmillan.
Irvine, J. *et al.* (eds) (1979). *Demystifying Social Statistics*. London: Pluto Press.
McLeod, C.J. and Slodatski, A.N. (1978). 'How to find out: a guide to searching the nursing literature' *Nursing Times*, 74, No. 6, 21–3.
Plummer, Kenneth (1983). *Documents of Life*. London: Allen and Unwin.

9

Survey research: design and sampling

In this chapter we have in mind the sort of research that a practitioner might do in his or her own institution:

1 surveying the attitudes of the client population to a service;
2 comparing two groups of clients to see, e.g. whether the medical and care needs of elderly men are different from those of elderly women, or whether black families have different social-work needs from white ones (a sort of 'case-control study' of *social* needs);
3 trying to predict outcomes or looking for causal links (e.g. whether some forms of nursing care are more effective than others at achieving a desired end, or whether clients who make repeated use of a counselling service differ systematically from those who come once and then drop out).

We look at how respondents are selected, how questions or observation schedules are constructed (including the construction of attitude and personality scales), what problems for the interpretation of the data can usefully be anticipated at the design stage and the eventual use of questionnaires in the field.

The usual stages of survey design are:

1 Formulating the 'problem' or area of study as precisely as possible – probably after:
(a) reviewing the 'literature';
(b) a first 'pilot' stage of talking to potential respondents in a fairly open and unstructured way about the topic(s) of the survey, to get their ideas and some notion of the terminology they use;
(c) where the research is to be carried out in a limited number of settings (e.g. one or a few institutions), spending some time there familiarizing yourself with what goes on.
2 Selecting the sample of respondents or settings, or devising rules for how a sample is to be picked.
3 Deciding on the best mode of 'delivery' – whether you are going to observe

behaviour in a systematic way or ask questions and, if you decide on a questionnaire, whether it will be administered by an interviewer or sent by post for self-completion or delivered by some other means. At this time you would plan what to do about refusals and non-response – whether and when to send 'follow-up' letters, for instance, and whether it is possible to collect any descriptive information about people who refuse to co-operate.

4 Thinking carefully about what descriptive ('demographic') information might be necessary or useful – age, gender, social class, etc. – and precisely how to record it.

5 Thinking what alternative explanations might be offered for any results you obtain, and what extra information you need to collect to explore them.

6 Designing the questionnaire or observation schedule. If this includes measurement scales not in common use, a second stage of pilot work would be needed, to check on the *validity* of the measures (looking for evidence that they do measure what you want) and their *reliability* (that they produce fairly stable and consistent results).

7 In a final pilot stage you would try out the questionnaire or schedule, to identify and deal with problems in its administration. You would also, at this stage, think about how the results are to be analysed, to make sure the date will be recorded in a suitable form.

These stages are described with the usual 'cross-sectional' survey in mind – wanting to know what is the case at present and asking a sample of people about it in a 'one-shot' survey design. When looking, for example, at changes over time, more sophisticated designs may be required, because of problems of memory and how the present tends to 'reconstruct' the past (see Chapter 6). The two classic ways round this kind of problem are:

1 repeated cross-sections – drawing fresh samples at each time-period, and asking about the present, e.g. sampling a population before TV becomes available, sampling it again afterwards, and comparing the two sets of results;

2 'panel' or 'cohort' designs – taking a group of people and asking them questions at designated time-periods, e.g. taking a sample before TV becomes available and questioning the *same* people again afterwards.

(We tend to talk of 'cohort studies' where the sample purports to be representative of an age-group, and otherwise of 'panel studies'.) The latter is superior in design terms, but more difficult to set up and maintain.

Most of this chapter will be about questionnaires – asking people questions about themselves and what they think and believe. We should start off by pointing out, however, that surveys do not *have* to ask people questions. The systematic observation of behaviour is an equally important survey technique, and where it is applicable it may be a stronger approach than verbal questioning, because you do not have the difficulty of interpreting the sense which respondents have made of the questions and what they meant by their answers. As a survey technique, observation must be *systematic* – it must entail counting or measuring behaviours in some consistent and reliable fashion. If you have to construct a classification system for yourself, your research would be preceded by a period of more general observation, to obtain a list of the behaviours which can be observed and to work out ways of defining them tightly. Often one researcher will devise a 'coding system' and have it tried out by other researchers; if they can also apply it consistently, then the system is a reasonably reliable one and not just the exteriorization of its author's fancies and prejudices. A further period of observation would then follow, in which all those who were destined to use the system practised it, preferably together and on the same 'cases', until a consistent level of performance emerged; this stage of training and practice would be equally necessary even if you were using another researcher's classification system. A better stratagem is to video the behaviour and do the classification afterwards. This lets you work over the same scene several times, with colleagues, until you reach agreement about what is going on.

Selecting respondents

The ideal 'sample survey' is a census – questioning every member of a population (every nurse or patient in a hospital, every client on the case-load, every household in an area). This is seldom practical, however, and so researchers have to *sample* their populations. Very many of the surveys of opinion with whose results we are bombarded by newspapers and manufacturers, however, are grounded in quite inadequate samples. Market researchers, for example, may ask their questions of people who pass in the city street, generally during the day. Such people are not typical of the population as a whole: they are those who happen to be on the street at the time, and probably under-represent people in full-time employment, people at schools or colleges, people who shop locally rather than in the city centre, and so on. Alternatively, they sometimes go from house to house in selected streets. This is a better stratagem, provided that all times of the day and days of the week are covered, but if not then they are again unlikely to draw representative samples, because they will exclude those who are not present at the time in question. Newspaper 'surveys' are often based on even less representative 'volunteer' samples – those who bother to answer a request for information, or those who write spontaneously about something that excites or annoys them. There are better ways of working than these – methods more likely to generate samples which are representative of their populations.

Random sampling

The best kind of sample for survey work is the *random* sample – one drawn from a complete list of the population (i.e. of those to whom we want the results to generalize) in such a way that every member of it has an equal chance of being represented and it is chance that determines which particular members are selected. A sample drawn in this way cannot be seen as influenced by the views and expectations of the researcher – you cannot pick a random sample deliberately in such a way as to 'prove' your own views – and, provided it is fairly large, it stands a good chance of resembling the population from which it is drawn. So if you were looking at some characteristics of your clients, a very good way to proceed would be to obtain a complete list of the current population of clients or of people who have come in over the past months or years, if the population is small, put all the names in a box, shake it well and draw out as many cases as you want for your sample. If the population is larger than that, you might want to take every nth name, from a randomly chosen starting point – for example, every tenth name, if you wanted a sample of 100 from a population of 1000.

Better still is to resort to a table of random numbers. These are published in all sets of statistical tables and most statistics textbooks, and they consist essentially of a string of numbers with no discernible pattern to them – e.g. 31415873920408279 . . . They may be arranged in sets of five or ten, in columns down the page. All you need to know, to pick a sample using them, is the size of your population and the desired size of sample. Say your population was 10 000, and you wanted a sample of 100. If you picked every hundredth case (as 10 000/100 = 100) you would get the right size of sample, but there might be some pattern to which cases came up a hundred apart – and if the population were actually 10 030, the last thirty cases would stand no chance at all of being selected. So you can use the first four numbers in the table to determine a random starting point: if they were 0001, you would start with the first case, but in this case they are 3141, so you start with the 3141st. Now you could take every hundredth case. Cleverer still is to divide up the population into hundreds and take the nth case from each hundred according to the next pair of random numbers – the 58th from the first hundred, the 73rd from the next hundred, and so on. (When you get to the last case on the list, you carry on counting from the beginning again, as if the cases were arranged in a circle.) This kind of procedure gives you absolutely the least chance of picking a sample which is in any way systematically biased.

If there is no complete list of the population, you might be able to draw a sample by taking the next n cases to come in (e.g. the next 50 cases, if you want a sample of 50), provided cases come in randomly and there is no systematic pattern to the order in which they are received. This last point is crucial, however, and you need to think very carefully about the possibility of patterns occurring – to use your researcher's imagination to think what might be happening. If you took the next 50 cases to come in to the casualty department of a hospital, for example, and you picked the period just after a disputed football match, you would get a very different sample from one drawn in the days immediately preceding Christmas (more victims of fights in the former case, and more victims of drunken driving in the latter). Different kinds of cases come in at night than during the day. It would clearly be best, if you want a representative sample, to pre-select times of the day, days of the week and weeks of the year, randomly, and use these as your 'collection points'. Wherever there is any possibility of patterns occurring in a population list or a series of admissions, you should make sure that your selection procedures are random enough to overcome it, and there is no single and simple way of doing so.

Because the random sample *is* random, drawn by chance, it is reasonably likely to be roughly representative of the population, but only roughly. It is possible to improve the representation by a process known as *stratification* – separately sampling the strata or layers of the population, using a variable known to be of some importance. If you draw a random sample of a year's hospital admissions, for example, there is every likelihood that your sample will be roughly representative of the population in terms of numbers of males and females, but only roughly. If you know that gender is an important variable in terms of your research question, you can improve the representative nature of your sample in this respect by drawing separate samples of males and females, in numbers proportionate to the numbers of the two in the population.

Cluster sampling

Frequently, when drawing samples from 'the world at large', rather than a particular institution or setting, a random sample is not appropriate because there is no list of the population from which to draw it, or because the geographical spread of a true random sample would be too great for a given researcher to handle. A random sample of 500 housewives scattered across the British Isles would not give more than one or two in each town, and a national random sample of schoolchildren or hospital patients would not be much more accessible. Here we often resort to a process called *cluster sampling* – picking geographical clusters, then sampling within them. If you wanted a national sample of hospital patients, for example, you might pick five or ten hospitals at random and then take a sample of patients within the sampled hospitals. If you wanted a sample of the people in a town, you might pick three or four districts at random, and within them three or four streets, and within them three or four houses, and then interview all the people in the designated houses. There is a risk that your sample will be unrepresentative because the range is constricted – if certain sorts of people occur according to some geographical pattern, then you may over-sample those sorts of people and under-sample other sorts. However, you can apply the principle of stratification to overcome this risk by selecting your clusters according to some sensible system. If you were sampling within a town, for example, you would make sure to pick some inner-urban areas and some suburban ones, and to select a mix of working-class areas and middle-class ones. If you were sampling hospitals, you would make sure that all types of hospital were represented.

Quota sampling

When nothing else is practicable we tend to resort to *quota sampling*. This is a procedure where we seek to obtain a representative sample of the population by setting up 'quotas', by sets of important variables, which match the population. We might set out, for example, to interview so many elderly middle-class women, so many elderly middle-class men, so many middle-aged middle-class women, and so on. This procedure will guarantee that the sample is representative with respect to the variables which are used to form the quotas. However, there is no control over other variables – interviewers may select whom they like to fill the quotas provided that the quota design is adhered to. Quite serious biases can, therefore, creep into the sampling. For example, in an Open University student survey (see Abbott and Sapsford 1987a) the student interviewers were set a quota design by age, social class and gender, and they matched it fairly exactly. However, the respondents whom they interviewed turned out overall to be better educated than the average, there were substantially more women in full-time employment than one would expect, and women in routine non-manual work were somewhat underrepresented. This pattern undoubtedly reflects the kinds of people Open University students find easy to locate and interview.

There are a number of ways in which quota sampling can be improved, if the interviewer is prepared to expend the effort. For example, an additional element of stratification may be introduced into samples of households by sampling from a variety of areas rather than allowing the quota to be filled from a single area. Time-periods can be randomized or systematically sampled, to minimize the risk of missing certain kinds of people because of their hours of work. A random element can be introduced – picking streets or postcodes at random as starting points. Nevertheless, and with all these improvements, quota sampling remains inherently inferior to random sampling as a way of guaranteeing a sample representative of its population.

It remains a widely used procedure in market research, however, because of its comparative ease and cheapness: there is no need for a complete list of the population to act as a sampling frame, and interviewers do not need to call back if they find a given respondent not at home, but can replace him or her with someone else of the right characteristics. In political opinion research quota sampling has almost entirely replaced more random methods because it has been found that the improvement of prediction given by the latter is too slight in this area of research to justify the extra cost (see McKee 1981).

Exercise 27: Sampling

The first six pages of your telephone directory will be the population for this exercise (or some other list with at least two hundred names on it). Count the number of names overall, and also (a) how many of the names have the letter 'a' as the second or third letter of the main word of the entry, and (b) how many of the entries are commercial or business addresses of some sort. Then take two types of samples:

1 do the same counts for the first 50 names in the list;
2 do the same counts for a random sample of 50 drawn using a table of random numbers.

Compare the results. Which type of sample comes closest to matching the population?

Devising the questions

If you are asking questions rather than observing behaviour, you need a questionnaire. (This holds even if you are interrogating not people, but files or documents; you still need a consistent list of questions to ask about them and a consistent way of recording the answers.) This will contain, broadly, three sorts of questions.

1 There will be demographic questions – age, gender, occupational details (for coding social class), and other explanatory or descriptive variables about people's lives that you are going to need at the analysis stage, such as where they live, the level of their education, etc. You will probably *pre-code* these – work out the possible range of answers and set up categories with the question, so that all that has to be done is to ring a number or tick a box. Be careful, however, to ensure:
   (a) that all possible answers are covered (you may need categories for 'don't know' and/or 'refused to answer');
   (b) that categories do not overlap (age is coded, e.g. as 20–29, 30–39, etc., not 20–30, 30–40, etc., because in the latter coding scheme the code for someone aged 30 is ambiguous); and
   (c) that you will get a reasonably even distribution of responses between the categories of a variable.
   If you do not know the age distribution of your population in advance, for example, it is better to record the actual age in years (or even years and months, for children) and work out categories afterwards.
2 Factual questions about people's past histories: whether they have been burgled in the past, when and for what they have been in hospital, their work histories, or whatever. The two problems here, both aspects of validity of measurement, are (a) definition and (b) memory. It is of paramount importance that you define precisely what you mean by the event or happening on which your respondents are to report; otherwise, differences between groups may be due to differences of interpretation, not differences of experience. Secondly, memory for the past is unreliable; people usually remember *what* has happened to them, but often not precisely *when*. So it is unwise to ask how many times x has happened 'in the last year'; precisely anchored time-periods such as 'since Christmas' are to be preferred.
3 Questions about attitudes and beliefs. These are more complex than they may at first appear, and there are several ways of proceeding. We shall talk about them in the next section.

Measuring attitudes

Much survey research is concerned with the measurement of attitudes, beliefs, opinions, intentions, etc. If you think of attitudes as something a person has and can report on, then the best way of getting at them is quite simply to ask about them. Much market research takes this stance: 'Which of these two coffees do you prefer?', 'Which would you buy, if they were the same price?' Much political research does likewise: 'How would you vote if there were a general election tomorrow?' The Abbott and Payne survey which we examined in Section 2 asked straightforwardly for people's opinions about hospital visiting and their preferences, as well as about their factual experiences. The only technical problem, in this approach, is to phrase the questions clearly, unambiguously and in such a way that the answers can readily be understood by the researcher.

Another view of the area of attitudes/beliefs/intentions would be to regard an attitude as something that a person has, but is not necessarily able to report – a complex of beliefs and tendencies to behave in certain ways, bound together from an outsider's point of view, but not necessarily apparent to the insider's conscious thought-processes. In that case you would want to find or construct some sort of 'measuring instrument'. You would administer a list of questions which can be shown to be 'symptomatic' of the attitude in question in a number of people, and add the answers together in some way to give a score. Many clinical scales are of this kind: they seek to measure a mental state (e.g. depression) by asking a number of relatively innocuous questions which people who have that particular state typically answer in one way – e.g. 'Do you often feel unhappy?', 'Do you often cry for no reason?', 'Do you have difficulty in sleeping?'. You might want to adopt this tactic if the question which underlies your scale is a sensitive one which might offend the respondent, or if there are very strong social norms prompting the respondent to answer in a particular direction.

One way of constructing such a scale is to get a panel of experts in the area in question to generate a pool of statements which they would see as symptomatic of the attitude or mental state, and use the ones on which the experts appeared to agree. A second and more common way of proceeding is to generate a large pool of items which have 'face validity' – they look at least as if they *ought* to measure what is required. You then go through at least four stages of pilot work.

1 You administer the items to a group of people (about 20?), getting them to score them on a 7-point scale from, for example, 'very true of me' to 'not at all true of me'. You throw out all those items which tend to attract scores in the middle of the scale from everyone, because they will not help to discriminate any group from any other.

2 You administer the remaining items to two separate groups who can be guaranteed to differ from each other on the variable which the scale is measuring – for example, if you were measuring 'satisfaction with the service we provide' you might pick 10 people who have taken the trouble to come and tell you afterwards how good the service was and the 10 people who had complained most virulently. You would keep the items which are consistently answered one way by one group and

the other by the other on average, throwing out those items which did not discriminate.

3 You would retest your original group, a little time afterwards, to see if they gave similar answers (a test of reliability).

4 You would validate the final scale by finding two more groups who undoubtedly differed on the variable in question and seeing if the scale differentiated between them (to ensure that you are not just capitalizing on a chance set of differences in the first pair of groups).

If you had professional resources at your disposal there are two more things you might well do:

5 You might get scores from a large sample of the normal population and from large samples of people who would be expected to score particularly high or low, to establish the normal range of scores and what might be expected of extreme groups.

6 Taking this fairly large data-set, you might subject it to *factor analysis*, a statistical procedure which tests whether all the items correlate together (the extent to which they are measuring the same thing) or whether one can distinguish groups of items which correlate with others within the group, but less so with items outside the group (in which case your scale may be measuring more than one variable).

The final scale is demonstrably valid and reliable. To the extent that these stages have not been undertaken, this cannot be asserted.

Yet another way of looking at attitudes, beliefs and intentions is to see them as products of how the respondent sees the world – what sort of a world he or she thinks we live in, with respect to your area of interest. One can get at people's ways of classifying their world, their 'constructs', by a technique devised by the American psychologist George Kelly (e.g. 1955), known as the Role Repertory Grid. This was originally devised for therapeutic interviews, but has since been widely used for a range of psychological studies of people and how they see the world, and even in market research (to explore 'brand images'). For an introduction to Kelly's theories and to uses of the Grid, see Bannister and Fransella (1971). A related technique is the semantic differential scale pioneered by Osgood *et al.* (1967), where sets of *supplied* adjectives form the scales on which people, groups or objects of interest are to be rated. The adjectives typically include some of very general reference (e.g. warm/cold, strong/weak) and perhaps some more specific to the particular research topic. You saw this technique in action in the Dingwall and Fox paper which we considered in Section 2.

Finally, a useful way of getting at difficult concepts unobtrusively is by the use of what are known as 'projective techniques' – segments of 'verbal behaviour' into which respondents may be seen as projecting or expressing some aspect of mentality. One classic, for example, is the TAT (Thematic Apperception Test), which consists of a series of ambiguous pictures looking something like magazine illustrations. The respondent is asked to write or narrate the story illustrated by each picture, and it is argued that what appears in the story (not being supplied by the pictures, which are as near neutral in content as possible) expresses something about the respondent. For example, a picture of two men in a room might be seen as brothers at home, or as two colleagues conspiring, or as a homosexual affair, or two people planning to start a successful small business, or . . . The original use of this test was to measure 'achievement motivation' by the amount of achievement-orientated imagery that was produced (McClelland *et al.* 1953). Another example would be the use of photographs to measure affective flattening – getting people to describe what they saw in pairs of photographs of people, and seeing the extent to which they did or did not impute emotions to the subjects of them (Dixon 1967; Sapsford 1983).

Anticipating problems

Non-response

Nearly all surveys have a problem of non-response: people refuse to answer, or randomly chosen respondents cannot be contacted, or if you left questionnaires to be filled in by the respondents some of them will not bother to do so. It would be very destructive of a survey's claims to represent the views of a population if the non-response rate were very large, and particularly if the non-respondents were not a random subset of the sample – if particular kinds of people tended not to respond. There is a certain amount you can do about this problem at the fieldwork stage and we shall discuss this later. Two precautions can be taken at the design stage, however. First, it may be possible to anticipate which kinds of people may not respond and to over-sample them: in a questionnaire about the banning of smoking at work, for example, you might deliberately set out to question more smokers than would be needed to represent their proportion of the population, anticipating that many smokers will be hostile to the purpose of the questionnaire. (This assumes, of course, that you know the population distribution and that you can reliably identify smokers and non-smokers beforehand.) This kind of *disproportionate stratification* is also useful for making sure that rare groups in the population are adequately represented. The second tactic is to try to find out at least basic demographic characteristics even of the non-responders, so that you can compare them with the respondents and see if they differ in any significant way. If you are interviewing face to face it should be possible to note gender and estimate age and even rough social class. If you are sending out questionnaires and ensuring confidentiality by *not* asking for names and addresses to be sent in, you might still get postcode or area of town on the respondents' questionnaires, and if you kept a note of how many you despatched to each post code or area of town then you can at least see if there is any geographical inequality in the response. (A directory of postcodes is kept in every central post office.)

Reactivity

A second problem which must be anticipated at the design stage is reactivity – the risk that some of the answers will be prompted by the way the questionnaire is designed or delivered. You will take great pains at the design stage, for example, to avoid social desirability effects – the tendency of people to 'be in favour of honour and virtue', and to give answers that will represent them as respectable and socially conforming in the eyes of the researcher – by finding ways of phrasing questions which allow the socially less unacceptable responses to seem acceptable. You will avoid too many questions which could naturally be answered 'yes' or 'no'. You would be very sure not to suggest in your question-working what answer you expect the informant to give. You would also be careful of the order of questions, so that the answer to one question is not suggested by the answer to a previous one.

Alternative explanations

Finally, you need to collect a certain number of demographic variables to test for whether they provide alternative explanations for your results to the explanation which you propose to put forward. If you were examining the relationship between unemployment and certain kinds of 'health behaviour', for example, it might be that poverty provided a more comprehensive explanation than unemployment – that all people in poverty showed the behaviour in question, whether or not they were registered as unemployed. You would, therefore, need to collect some kind of measure of household income, to check whether this was the case. You would also want to collect the obvious demographic characteristics – age, gender, social class, etc. – in order to be able to check that your sample *is* typical of the population.

Exercise 28: Questionnaire design

Try your hand at designing a questionnaire. Imagine you are commissioned to examine clients'/patients'/customers' satisfaction with the service your agency or firm provides (if you work for an agency or firm), or with a service which you or your family receive (e.g. the service provided by your local primary school). Think carefully what this 'service' is – how many different things the agency or firm does, and the different goals which the clients, etc., might have. (You may need to talk to some people before you start.) Think also who the clients actually are – in the case of a school, for example, are the clients children, or parents, or the education authority or all of these? Then work out what questions you need to ask, including demographic variables for describing the population, checking on the quality of the sampling and looking for patterns in the results. (You may need different questionnaires for the different kinds of 'client', if their interests are different.) Think carefully *how* you would ask the questions, for maximum acceptability to the respondents and maximum clarity when you come to analyse the results. If you are able, try your draft out on three or four appropriate people, and see what changes you want to make to it after you have seen their responses.

Doing the research

An essential element of research design which we have not yet discussed (because it affects fieldwork even more than design) is the notional 'research contract' between you and your respondents. You will, of course, have ensured that your research procedures will not cause pain or distress to informants, but what are you going to tell them about the research? Are you asking questions to collect data, regarding what you do with the data as in a sense none of their business? Or are you adopting a fully collaborative stance, taking them fully into your confidence, carrying out the work as much to further their interests as your own and regarding the work as in some sense 'joint property'? If the latter, have you worked out what form the collaboration will take? Will they be collaborating in the writing of the report? Will they have free access to each other's data (see 'confidentiality', below)? If they disagree with your interpretation of the data, do they have the right to change what is reported, or to have their disagreement registered, or are their comments to be only advisory? If you enter into a collaboration, the rules must be clear to all parties.

It is general practice to promise respondents *confidentiality* – that only you will be able to match up names and questionnaires, and that the information will never be used in such a way that the respondent can be identified. You will need to think carefully about building in procedures which ensure that this is the case – for example, sampling widely enough that no individual is unique. Confidentiality is particularly important if the respondents stand to lose by being identified – if, for example, they are patients or clients of your agency, or working colleagues, and their views could be held against them by 'management'. (Sometimes respondents will not *want* confidentiality – when they want their specific complaints to be dealt with, for example.)

Also a design matter, as well as an aspect of fieldwork, is precisely how you intend to deliver the questionnaire. Will you take it round to respondents yourself and ask them the questions, filling in the answers yourself? Will you use other (perhaps paid) people as interviewers. Will you hand it out personally, but ask them to fill it in for themselves and return it to you? Or will you post it to them and ask them to return it? Each of these methods has advantages as well as disadvantages. If you are your own interviewer, you can have maximal confidence in the data. You will also probably get a fairly low refusal rate. On the other hand, you cannot cover very many cases. Postal delivery is the best method for reaching a wide target population, but the refusal/non-response rate is generally very high; 50 per cent response would be considered quite high for a postal survey. You will, therefore, do everything you can to increase response rate if you adopt the postal strategy: including a stamped addressed envelope for the return of the form, and writing again, perhaps two or three times, to people who do not respond to the first letter. (This is, of course, impossible unless you are sending the questionnaire to preselected named individuals.) Delivering the questionnaire yourself improves the response rate, but there are still problems. Finally, using others as your interviewers can give you the advantages of personal interviewing, but allow you to cover more cases than you could manage by yourself. It may, indeed, be the only way to obtain face-to-face interviews if you are not an appropriate person to be carrying out the interviews yourself. For example, it is better to have a black interviewer when approaching black people, and a young interviewer when approaching young people – respondents are more at their ease and less likely to give an 'official response'. On the other hand, it is very important that the interviewers be trained to use the questionnaire all in the same way; otherwise differences might be due to characteristics of the interviewers' behaviour rather than characteristics of the respondents.

This question of training also applies to you yourself, if you are administering your own questionnaire. The whole point of this approach is that data shall be collected in a uniform manner from all respondents – that they all answered the same questionnaire, administered in the same fashion. (This is another argument against postal delivery – that you cannot control the conditions under which the questionnaire is filled in.) It is quite vital that all who are to administer the questionnaire know exactly what to do with each question, including the extent to which it is legitimate to explain what is meant and the extent to which they may be required to prompt respondents for more information. The questionnaire must be as standardized a measuring instrument as a thermometer, if we are to put complete confidence in its results.

Finally, we cannot over-stress the importance of pilot work. All questionnaires should be tried out, to see what could go wrong, before being administered to the sample at large. It is particularly important to pilot questions, scales, etc., which are intended to measure aspects of attitude, intention or personality.

These are of little value as evidence if you cannot demonstrate they are reliable (answered the same way by the same informants over a period of time short enough that change would not be expected) and valid as measures of what you claim that they measure.

Further reading

Survey design

Marsh, C. (1982). *The Survey Method*. London: Allen and Unwin.
Polgar, Stephen and Thomas, Shane (1988). *Introduction to Research in the Health Sciences*. London: Churchill Livingstone.
Witts, L.J. (ed.) (1964). *Medical Surveys and Clinical Trials*. London: Oxford University Press.

Measurement scales and psychological/attitude tests

Anastasi, Anne (1982). *Psychological Testing*. London: Macmillan.
Hollander, Edwin (1981). *Principles and Methods of Social Psychology*. Oxford: Oxford University Press (Chapter 3).

Jensen, Arthur (1981). *Straight Talk about Mental Tests*. London: Macmillan.
Newmark, Charles (1985). *Major Psychological Assessment Instruments*. Boston: Allyn and Bacon.
Osgood, Charles *et al.* (1967). *The Measurement of Meaning*. Urbana; Illinois, University of Illinois Press.

Role repertory grids and George Kelly's approach

Bannister, Don and Fransella, Fay (1971). *Inquiring Man*. Harmondsworth: Penguin.
Kelly, George (1955). *The Psychology of Personal Constructs*. New York: Norton.

Quantitative (statistical) analysis

To teach statistics is beyond the scope of this book, but there are many good texts on the market. Two books are particularly recommended. The first is the best for the beginner, a very good introductory text; it was recommended to us by our students. The other is also good, and does not assume any prior knowledge of statistics, but it is pitched more at good third-year students and postgraduates.

Clegg, Frances (1982). *Simple Statistics*. Cambridge: Cambridge University Press.
Marsh, Catherine (1988). *Exploring Data*. Cambridge: Polity.

10

Experimental practice

In this chapter we shall assume that any experiment you want to carry out will be a 'field experiment', set in the real world. We shall look mainly at how you would go about evaluating some aspect of your own potential practice – how you would try out a new treatment technique or style of working. The same techniques would also be appropriate for wider-scale testing of new practices – for assessing the effects of a new management structure or a general change in practice imposed from outside, or for comparing wards or wings of an institution in which different regimes were in force. (You should note, however, that this kind of controlled trial is by no means the only way in which practices can be evaluated. Most of the rest of this book will be about evaluation, offering a wide range of styles of working. This chapter is firmly set within a positivist epistemology and is concerned more with demonstrating causal influences than with understanding the nature of phenomena.)

Action research

The simplest kind of 'experimental' research you can do is *action research* in its crudest form – making a change and seeing what happens. Though by no means the best design for the purpose, this is a very common form of research into practice, often used in circumstances where nothing more elaborate is possible or where insufficient preparation rules out better designs. To obtain interpretable results, careful and reliable measurement and exhaustive documentation are essential. We need a clear and reliable measurement or description of what the treatment procedure or programme of change *is*, so that we know what it is that is causing any change that may occur. We need a clearly defined set of outcome measures, so that we can see what change is brought about. We need also to measure anything in the environment which might function as an alternative explanation of the results.

Measurement of the treatment and the outcome are not as simple as might at first appear. We need to have thought very carefully about what it is we are trying to achieve and what will count as having achieved it. In psychiatric and counselling research, for example, it is seldom possible to produce definitive proof of 'cure' following treatment – something that would be accepted by others, rather than just the researcher's/therapist's personal judgement. One tends, therefore, to ask the clients/patients what they *thought of* the therapy and whether they were satisfied with it; at least this is something more concrete than the therapist's judgement of his or her own cases. However, whether a feeling of satisfaction in the patient or client is what the therapist was trying to achieve is open to question: would he or she not be better satisfied with an amelioration of the condition, whether or not the patient felt good about the therapy. There is a great tendency in experimental research to substitute something measurable but not totally appropriate for the outcome which we really want to assess. If you were carrying out the research for someone else, you would need to think even more carefully about what outcome is desired and not necessarily to accept what the client *said* was the outcome. A declared aim of a hospital administration, for example, might be to improve the care of certain patients, as measured perhaps by whether they had to be re-admitted for the same condition within a specified time-period. However, it is a reasonable bet that they would not implement a recommendation to increase staffing levels unless it could be shown that the costs of re-admission were higher than those of increasing the intensity of nursing care.

Reactivity is the second problem. Inevitably, your ideas about the measurement of effectiveness have an effect on your practice – you do such and such because it appears to be working. We have hinted at this already, talking about problems in defining output measures: it is essential that you define what shall count as a success *before* starting to measure. Otherwise you are in the position of the punter who placed his bet after the race was won: you are claiming to predict what you have, in fact, observed happening. The nature of the treatment itself is even more prone to reactive effects in this kind of research. To the extent that you are not able to define precisely what your treatment will be *before* starting to measure its effects, your results will always be suspect: you may always have modified what you are doing to fit in with changes which you have observed (unconsciously, even). There will also be *confounded variables* – factors associated with your treatment which might provide alternative explanations of the outcome. In the earlier part of this century, great claims were made for the efficacy of insulin injections as a cure for certain kinds of mental disorder. These claims were dispelled by later analysis of what the process entailed – extreme physical debilitation, followed during the recovery period by constant and sympathetic attention from nurses. The subsequent discovery that the attention and sympathy were equally effective when *not* accompanied by the insulin injection more or less put paid to this therapy's claims.

The problem is in three parts.

1 There will be aspects to what you are doing of which you are not aware –
  probably aspects of your own behaviour and the way you budget your
  time.
2 These may as easily explain any changes which you observe as the deliberate manipulation of treatment which you are instituting.
3 There may be no way, within the crude design of this kind of action
  research, of separating out these effects: doing a certain kind of therapy or
  social work or nursing care may inevitably mean spending more time with
  the 'experimental' subjects or behaving to them in a certain kind of way,
  and it may always be this rather than the deliberate manipulation which is
  producing the effect.

The best you can do is to try to note all these confounded influences –
perhaps, if possible, getting someone else to watch you at work and examine
your practice – and note them in your report as areas for further study.

Exercise 29: Critique of action research

Imagine you have just joined the staff of a ward or office where a new procedure has
been introduced. What steps would you take to monitor its progress. (Assume that
back records, etc., are not available.) More important, what could you *not* conclude
from your results. (Think of this as a logical problem, not a practical one.)

However well you design this kind of study, it has certain logical flaws which
inevitably mean that what can be concluded from it is strictly limited. You
may institute a change and observe a result. However:

1 you can never be quite sure what produced the result – all manner of things
  will have been changed by the fact of your instituting an 'experiment', apart
  from your nominated treatment or experimental manipulation;
2 there may have been differences between people which are equally responsible for who showed the 'effect', and while you may have collected information about these, your 'sample' will lack sufficient structure for you to be
  able to disentangle or disprove such effects by statistical means;
3 you will not be able to say whether the effect would have occurred even
  without the treatment;
4 worst of all, you will not even be able to specify what the effect *is* – you will
  have measurements on how people perform after the treatment, but in the
  design discussed so far you have nothing with which to compare them.

Towards the controlled trial

The easiest of the faults to remedy in this very crude model of action research is
the problem of knowing whether a change has occurred or not. The first and
most basic element in any experimental design is that measurement of the

dependent variable(s) shall be undertaken *before* the manipulation/treatment is undertaken as well as afterwards. Indeed, to do so would be characteristic of any decently planned action research. Your basic data, in looking for causal influences, are not measurements, but differences between measurements: we are looking, not for some absolute value of a dependent variable, but for a *change* in it. You might, indeed, go further; if what you have achieved is a lasting change, not just a temporary one, then you will need post-treatment measurements after a period of time to demonstrate the fact.

However, as we noted in Chapter 5, a series of measurements on one group which has received a treatment are not in themselves logically convincing. Certainly, you can demonstrate that a change has occurred, but you cannot demonstrate *why* it occurred. Specifically, you cannot demonstrate that it occurred as a result of the treatment which was applied; it may be due to any number of other things which occurred to the group being treated during the same time as the treatment. The other essential of experimental design, therefore, is a control or comparison group – one which is alike in every respect to the treatment group, and undergoes as similar as possible a set of experiences, but does not actually receive the treatment (in drug research they would typically receive a placebo or dummy – a pill or injection which looked like the experimental drug, but was in fact chemically inert). One basic stratagem for making sure that the two groups are alike is to assign people *randomly* to treatment and control groups, as we have seen: provided your groups are reasonably large, this should 'even out' any chance differences. Guaranteeing similarity of experience is more difficult, outside the laboratory, but you would want to document their lives in as much detail as possible during the period of the experiment, looking for any possibly significant differences.

As we pointed out in Chapter 5, there are other ways of picking control/comparison groups which may be more effective for some purposes. With small numbers you probably need to institute some kind of *matching* procedure, picking pairs of subjects who are comparable on variables which you know might well be important (age, class, gender, medical condition, social circumstances, or whatever) and allocating one of the pair at random to each group. This absolutely guarantees comparability at least on these variables. Indeed, where you are trying to control for some well known alternative explanation at the design stage matching is perhaps the best stratagem; like stratification in random sampling (see Chapter 9), it may improve on the simple random procedures in ways which are important to you. Best of all, if your design lends itself to it, is to use the same subjects as both 'experimentals' and 'controls': then you are certain that those in the two groups have the same history, the same physical and mental constitution, etc. This is seldom possible in practice, however, because the administration of the treatment alters the subjects to the point where they are no longer comparable with their past selves with regard to the manipulation which you want to test.

The allocation of subjects to treatment and control groups raises an important point about the conduct of experiments. It is for each researcher to decide whether the purity of including an untreated control group is worth the ethical dilemma of leaving some people deliberately untreated, but on the whole many researchers and professionals would regard doing so as unethical in a wide range of circumstances. A way round may be to compare a new treatment with people undergoing the best of what was previously available: then at least no-one has deliberately been debarred from treatment. It is often difficult to reconcile the needs of the research – including the benefit to future sufferers if a treatment can be shown unambiguously to 'work' – with the deliberate mis- or non-treatment of a proportion of sufferers.

A final point to watch is what is known as the *Hawthorne Effect*. The name derives from a famous series of studies at the Hawthorne Works in Chicago in the 1920s (Roethlisberger and Dickson 1939). The researchers were commissioned to seek ways of changing environment and working conditions to improve output, and they tried out a range of possible modifications each of which did, indeed, improve output – improving lighting and physical comfort, introducing coffee breaks, shortening the working day, etc. However, when as the last stage of the experiment (using a 'same-subjects' design) they returned everything to its original state, output went up again. It was concluded that the major (and confounded) variable, which might have been responsible for any of the results, was the subjects' awareness that they were taking part in an experiment. To the extent that the subjects of your treatment *know* that it is a new treatment, their reactions may be conditioned by this knowledge as much as by the treatment itself. Even your *own* knowledge that your treatment is experimental may change your behaviour in unconscious ways, enough that how you behave is not how you would behave if the new procedure had been accepted and you were applying it routinely. Drug researchers commonly adopt what is called a 'double-blind' technique, where neither the recipient of the drug nor the person handing it out in conformity with a pre-arranged administration schedule knows whether what is received is the active drug or an inactive placebo. The ethics of this kind of procedure in social research may again be open to question, however.

Exercise 30: Experiment

Try making some small change in your own practice: a change of procedures or the ordering of jobs, aimed at getting patients to talk to each other more, or a different way of arranging your interviews with people to set them apparently more at their ease, or a different way of budgeting your time to allow more time for study or to get the household chores over faster. Think carefully, before you start, what precisely your manipulation or treatment is to be – write it out as a set of instructions for yourself – and what is to count as having achieved your desired outcome (in measurable terms). Think what other changes might occur as a result of your changed behaviour, which might affect the outcome, and think about ways of measuring these and controlling for them either in the design or statistically at the stage of analysis. Start your measurements before you start your 'treatment', to give yourself a baseline 'before' measure with which your outcome can be compared. Think carefully also about the extent to which the fact that it is your own practice which you are examining may contaminate the results. For example, to what extent might the awareness of an impending experimental change affect your behaviour during the period of measurement before the experiment started?

Quasi-experimental logic

A sure way of getting over most ethical problems with experimental research is the 'natural experiment' or 'quasi-experimental comparison' (the 'case-control study' of medical research). Here what you do is to take a change which is being imposed anyway and collect or obtain statistics from before the change, during it and after it. These are treated as the 'pre-test' and 'post-test' statistics of the true experiment. You can generally organize some kind of control or comparison group as well: a similar area in which the change is not occurring, for example. A classic example is the Connecticut Crackdown, a change in motoring laws in one American state which was aimed at decreasing traffic fatalities. A team of researchers looked at the changes it made to fatality statistics by comparing figures from before the changes of law and practice to figures from after it (Campbell and Ross, 1968; Ross and Campbell, 1968; Campbell, 1969). They controlled for extraneous events by comparing surrounding states, where these changes had not been made, and found that fatalities did not decrease similarly over the same period. The argument that it was the changes in law and practice which brought about the change in death-rate is, therefore, fairly convincing, and the logic of the argument follows the argument of an experiment. Its weakness, however, is that the design is *not* experimental in that there is no control over allocation to experimental and control groups. However carefully the two are matched, it is always possible to argue that there may be some unobserved difference between the two which is responsible for the results.

Finally, two points which we have made earlier in the book are worth repeating here, because they have implications for your own design of research:

1 The basic purpose of many pieces of survey research is quasi-experimental comparison – looking for the association of one variable with another, with the intention of arguing about causal influence. This is why it is so important to pre-guess alternative explanations and collect variables relevant to them, to be able to eliminate them by statistical control at the analysis stage.
2 On the other hand, many studies which masquerade as true experiments are at best quasi-experimental, because there is no true control over allocation to groups. Experiments comparing males and females, for example, are at best quasi-experimental: there may be characteristics contingently associated with gender, but not central to its definition – such as experience of early socialization, for example, or outright discrimination and stereotyping in adult life – which are confounded with gender itself and cannot be eliminated by any kind of random allocation. The same holds true for experiments comparing clinical types, or different types of offender, or any

experiments where the allocation to groups rests in essence on a 'naturally' occurring difference.

Further reading

Breakwell, Glynnis *et al.* (eds) (1982). *Social Psychology: A Practical Manual.* London: Macmillan/British Psychological Society.

Polgar, Stephen and Thomas, Shane (1988) *Introduction to Research in the Health Sciences.* London: Churchill Livingstone.

Witts, L.J. (ed.) (1964). *Medical Surveys and Clinical Trials.* London: Oxford University Press.

$$\equiv 11 \equiv$$

Open interviewing

This chapter deals with the conduct of 'open' or 'unstructured' interviews with groups of people. You might be interviewing simply to find out people's views on a topic or a service, not knowing enough in advance to put together a structured questionnaire. (Indeed, a short phase of open interviewing is a normal precursor to constructing a questionnaire – 'mapping the ground', finding out the range of views and topics which should be covered, learning the language in which informants are likely to express themselves.) You might be exploring a topic where it is desirable not to introduce previous theory, but to 'let the participants speak for themselves'. Much feminist work is of this kind, trying not to apply preconceived (and male-conceived) categories to women's lives, but talking to them to see what *they* think is important and how *they* understand their world. You might be carrying out an evaluation of a setting or of a service you have been providing, and need to get at how the clients and staff have experienced it without letting your own or management's preconceptions intrude. You might be doing something much less structured – talking to groups of people who fall in categories of interest, just to understand their lives and how they make sense of them.

'Open interviewing' is not one method, but our term for a range of different ways of proceeding. They have in common:

1 the aim of eliciting the informants' views in the informants' own terms;
2 the attempt to make the interviews resemble natural conversations as far as possible;
3 the desire to impose as little as possible of the researchers' ideas on the conversation.

While agreeing on these aims, however, interviewers have differed a great deal over how to pursue them. Some interviews are virtually undirected by the researcher, with the informant controlling most of the direction of the conversation. In others the interviewers take more control, trying to cut through 'irrelevance' and 'keep the informant to the point'. Most inter-viewers go in with an outline 'agenda', but for some this consists only of a list of topic areas to cover and a few 'stock questions' to get things started and bridge gaps in the conversation. In other cases, however, the researcher may have a quite detailed list of questions to ask of all informants and may even try to determine the order in which they are answered. Mostly, we adopt a 'neutrally sympathetic' manner when interviewing, but in some research (e.g. on managers of large corporations) the researchers have thought it appro-priate to adopt an adversarial style and provoke an argument in order to test the informants' beliefs. All of these are valid ways of doing interview research, and each has its strengths and corresponding weaknesses. On the whole, the more structured the approach, the less the naturalism and the more the danger of attributing the researchers' ideas to the informants. On the other hand, structure makes for uniformity of coverage and so for more interpretable data.

We work backwards in this chapter, from the nature of the work to the ways in which it is conducted. What kind of an exercise you think you are undertaking – what model you hold of the informants and their social world – shapes not only the analysis of the data, but also the conduct of the interviews and the way the study is initially planned, so this is considered first. Thereafter, we talk about the conduct of interviews, about gaining access to informants and about the selection of informants.

The nature of the data

At its simplest, the open interview is a way of finding out what people *think* about a situation. With the minimum of imposed structure necessary to keep the focus of the interview within bounds and save ourselves the time involved in listening to totally extraneous material, we let people talk about the situa-tion and what matters to them about it. This is by far the best way of finding out what is *salient* to them about it – what most readily springs to their lips. With a little probing to get them to assess which ideas matter and which are just 'tried on' to see how well they hold together in the interview situation, we can assess what is *central* – what they see as the irreducible core of their beliefs. We would probably impose an agenda of areas to be covered, so that we can be sure all informants have covered the same ground. We should be careful how we used such an agenda, however, or our introduction of particular topics could obscure whether they were, in fact, salient for the particular informant; once we have introduced a topic, we can no longer tell whether it would have cropped up spontaneously in the course of the interview.

An alternative view of how people work and make sense of their world is to see them as not always aware of what is important to them. If we want to know what the informant *feels* – what motivates his or her behaviour, whether or not he or she is aware of it or able (or willing) to mobilize it in conversation – then we must see our task in a rather different way. People may well have a set of well articulated views – a 'rhetoric' – which are strongly held and firmly believed, but their actual behaviour and the decisions they make may sometimes suggest to the outsider a quite different set of norms and values. For example, the more educated respondents generally have a clear and consistent set of beliefs to enunciate about social class, the structure of society and their place in it. When it comes to asking them about the detail of their lives, however – which schools their children go to and why they are 'good' or 'bad', which areas they see as good or bad ones to live in and why, to what kinds of job they aspire for their children and why – an equally clear set of implicit beliefs often emerges, but one which is not consistent with their declared 'rhetorical' position. This matter of rhetoric is an important one for open interviewing: whether we accept what the informant says at face value, or allow that we may all have sets of verbal beliefs which are sincerely held, but which may *not* be the unifying principles behind our practical actions.

If you hold this view of how people work in the social world, then you will be imposing a little more structure on the occasion than if you just accept what informants say at face value. You will be introducing questions, and areas of discussion, precisely in order to 'get underneath' the rhetoric and see what you can elicit about the less formally organized and recognized structuring principles which people apply to the social world when making their practical decisions. Doing so, however, will face you with the ethical question of the extent to which you are prepared to 'lead informants on' in order to elicit from them material which it is your intention to interpret in ways which might well offend them.

Now suppose that what you are trying to find out is what the informants *want done about* a situation – how to solve a problem which has occurred, or how to improve an institutional setting, say. A mixture of these two 'models' would undoubtedly be what is appropriate. You would be required and require yourself to represent faithfully the views which the participants had expressed. At the same time you might suspect that the immediate focus of complaint was not really 'what was wrong', and so you would be looking beyond and underneath their 'rhetoric' for more nebulous features of their situation which might be at fault. If you were playing your research to any extent collaboratively – as seems wise and reasonable, if there were any chance of your 'solution' being foisted on the informants – then you would want to discuss your eventual conclusions with them and reshape them to reflect their reactions (perhaps several times, until you found a set of recommendations and a form of words for expressing them which was acceptable to all parties). Given courage, you might even discuss your conclusions about particular interviews with the individual participants, before coming to a public set of general conclusions. This would take courage, however, if you had presumed to any extent to 'see behind the words' and draw conclusions on the basis of knowing better than the informant what was important in his or her life.

Doing the interviews

The core of the open style of interviewing is a very lively appreciation of how you are trying to present yourself and the task and the way in which the informant is making sense of the task and of you (in a word, *reflexivity*). Right from the start of any such project you would be watching carefully whether you 'came across' in your professional identity (social worker, nurse, doctor), or as a student, or as a 'researcher' perhaps associated with an academic institution, or as someone writing a book, or whatever. You will be monitoring carefully the impression you give of the task – whether it is a student exercise, or the gratification of your own curiosity, or an academic investigation or a study of shortcomings that might perhaps be put right as a result of it. Who you are and what the task is seen to be is all the informants have out of which to make sense of the exercise, and what sense they make will crucially determine what kind of an account they give of the phenomena in which you are interested.

Your choice of location for the interview (if you have a choice!) will be governed by the principle of naturalism: you will try to put yourself and the interview in a 'frame' which might be a natural one for the informant. For many purposes the informant's own home may be the best setting – putting oneself in the territory of the other – but there are circumstances where the home might be the wrong context. Talking to people about their work, for instance, it may be better to talk at the work-place or, better still, wherever they go to relax after work sessions – the canteen, the staff room, the local public house. There may be circumstances where the interview is best conducted on your own territory – in your office, or at the bed-side – but this will generally be appropriate only if you normally ask questions or have conversations with that informant in that setting. Best of all, if you are doing more than one interview with the same person, may be to vary the setting and take note of the different shades of perspective which are expressed in the different settings.

In the interview itself you will be trying to present yourself as friendly, but neutral, as someone not intimately involved in any disputes or differences of interest which may be mentioned. If the conversation is to be at all natural and relaxed you will have to say a bit about yourself and to contribute opinions to the flow of the occasion. To the extent that it is possible, however, you will avoid doing so – even if you are adopting a collaborative stance and interviewing for a declared and agreed purpose. It is all too easy, reading the transcript of an interview after the event, to see where opinions or categorizations of your own have been taken up and incorporated by the informant, so that you cannot tell whether they are part of the way in which the informant sees the world or 'on loan' from the interviewer. It is regrettably all too easy to express your own attitude to a situation and have the respondent agree with you – perhaps out of conviction, but perhaps out of politeness or a desire to adopt a 'socially desirable point of view'. Insofar as is possible, in a situation which can only be what it is because of your participation in it, you must avoid these forms of reactivity by contributing as little as is feasible; it is the informant whose views and feelings you want to collect, not your own. To the extent that detachment is not possible, you must try to be aware of your own contribution, take notes on it immediately afterwards, and if necessary report on it in your account of the findings.

Before entering the field you will have taken the opportunity to read as much as you can about the background and circumstances of the people whom you will be interviewing. If you are to be working in a hospital, you will read anything that has been written on that hospital or that class of hospitals, including what is said about it in Parliament and in the newspapers, to get a feel for the 'working rules' and the declared aims, and to be aware of any outstanding problems (e.g. financial). If you are interviewing a particular class of professional staff, you will scan their professional journals for articles expressing their problems and discontents and for what you can find on the 'letter page'. If you are talking to a group of people who have a given medical condition, you will familiarize yourself with the literature on that condition. If you are talking to people who fall in a 'social problem' category, you will make sure you are familiar with the benefits and services available to such a group. When you go into the field you will want to be as well informed as possible, so that you do not miss veiled allusions to common features of the situation and so that you are aware of any glaring omissions in participants' accounts.

On the other hand, you will want to conceal your knowledge as far as possible. The correct role for the qualitative researcher has often been described as that of the 'amiable incompetent' – someone friendly and intelligent but lacking knowledge, someone who has to be *told* things. (This may pose ethical problems, when for instance you know of some benefit or service to which the informant is entitled, but which he or she has not claimed. Try to restrict the information which you yourself communicate to the end of interviews, so as not to contaminate the material you collect or to 'break role' more than is necessary.)

Two particular problems arise when you are yourself a known 'expert' – e.g. a health visitor interviewing other health visitors. The first is that it is difficult to get your informants to 'spell things out', because they assume you must know all about it already. The other and more serious is that you will find it difficult to put aside your professional socialization and 'make the familiar strange' – to ask your informants to spell out what they mean rather than filling in the gaps from your own knowledge. This matters because your knowledge may, in fact, be faulty: informants may not mean what you take for granted that they mean, and they may not have shared precisely your professional experience.

How much you ask direct questions will depend on the time available and the subject of the interview. To get the best out of this approach you will want at least some early portion of the interview to be conducted in a fairly undirected fashion, letting the informant develop things at his or her pace and seeing what crops up without prompting. To be sure you have covered the topic which is of interest to you in enough detail that you can be sure of doing justice to your informant's views, however, you may have to resort to direct prompting, to explore topic areas that have not come up by themselves. Remember, however, that once a topic has been introduced by you, you can never know whether it would have come up spontaneously. Best practice if time permits might be to have more than one interview with each informant and to save direct prompts for later ones; then you could also introduce questions on views and topic areas which had not come up in the particular interview, but *had* been raised by another informant.

Selecting informants

While representative sampling is not and cannot be a major issue in this kind of work, because the sample size you will be able to handle is small, there is nonetheless every reason to try to pick 'cases' randomly from a sampling frame if at all possible, to avoid the charge of having deliberately chosen them to make a point or of having an unrealised bias in the sampling. In our mental handicap research (Abbot and Sapsford 1987b), for example, we were able to use the rolls of the 'special schools' as a sampling frame for families with a mentally handicapped child. There was no similar frame for the comparison group of families with no child bearing this label, however. What we did was to ask each interviewed mother for names and addresses of two or three other women on the same street or nearby who had a child of about the same chronological age as the mentally handicapped child, and how many other children they had. This enabled us to pick a comparison group who were roughly matched on geographical location (which was related to social class) and number of children. (We did not ask for introductions, preferring to make our own.) Sometimes personal introduction is the only way to put together a group for interview at all, if the criterion characteristic is a rare or concealed one – asking one example for names of others, asking *them* for further names, and continuing in this way until a sufficiently large group of interviews is achieved. This process is called *snowball sampling*, and it risks the obvious biases that you will only have access to 'cases' who know other 'cases', not to isolates, and that you may exhaust one part of the 'field' without ever encountering the other part. For example, in the mental handicap research a snowball sample which started with a mother whose child was at one type of special school might have given us a group of mothers from that school and none from the other school (which would have mattered, as the two schools dealt with cases of different severity). However, it may, on occasion, be the only way of proceeding.

A characteristic of an extended open interview project design is often the use of *theoretical sampling* – the selection of cases and groups, initially or as the research progresses, to explore aspects of the developing conclusions. In the mental handicap research, for example, we knew from the start that we would want to interview mothers of 'ordinary' children as well as mothers of mentally handicapped ones, to be able to distinguish problems of having a handicapped child from the general problems of having a child at all. If time and resources had allowed the research to continue further, we might have interviewed a group of mothers of physically handicapped children (to distinguish problems of *mental* handicap), or perhaps families caring for mentally handicapped adults (to distinguish problems associated with mentally handicapped *children*).

Gaining access

We have mentioned already the problem of 'gatekeepers'. Often it is necessary to 'get past' certain key figures before gaining access to the informants whom you want to interview. In a hospital you would need the permission of the administrative authorities, the co-operation of those in charge of wards and of other nursing staff, probably clearance from an Ethical Committee and so on. At each of these stages three things will be happening. First, you will be giving an account of your research, and this will undoubtedly be passed on, if only in a spirit of helpfulness and to prepare the ground for you. Your initial introduction to the setting will, therefore, be made not by you but by the gatekeepers. The second is that by having the permission or active co-operation of those in authority you may become identified with them in the eyes of the informants – particularly important in prison or school research, or in any setting where informants feel themselves controlled. You can do a certain amount to counteract these effects in your own initial introduction and in the course of the interviews, but you need to be alert for any differences they may have made to how you are perceived and what kinds of account you are being given. Such circumstances might be seen as a very good reason for interviewing each informant more than once, to try and build up an independent relationship of your own with them. The third effect will be that gatekeepers control to some extent whom you interview, steering you away from those who in their judgement are likely to be disturbed or harmed by the process. They may even steer you away from 'awkward cases' who would, in fact, make perfectly good informants, because in their judgement these people would not co-operate. There is not much you can do about this except to try to note that it has occurred.

During your discussions with gatekeepers, and during or immediately after your interviews, you will be taking reflexive notes of what is going on, what went wrong or went well, and how you and the task seem to be being understood. You will also want to take notes of any interaction between you and your informants occuring outside the frame of the interview. These will be needed at the analysis stage and to provide reliable reflexive material for the final report.

Exercise 31: Planning an open interviewing project

Suppose you were planning an interview project to explore the nature of the health visitor's job, how would you go about it? How would you set the project up, what kinds of people would you interview, and in what way?

Further reading

Burgess, Robert (1984). *In the Field*. London: Allen and Unwin.
Hammersley, Martyn and Atkinson, Paul (1989). *Ethnography: Principles in Practice*. London: Routledge.
McCracken, Grant (1988). *The Long Interview*. Beverly Hills: Sage.
Patton, Michael (1987). *How to Use Qualitative Methods in Evaluation*. Beverly Hills: Sage.

Answers to Exercise 31

When one of us (Abbott) undertook this kind of research, she conceptualized the purpose as 'to see how health visitors made sense of their professional role', in the light of literature which suggested that they themselves were uncertain about their role and its relationship to social work on the one hand and nursing on the other. She discussed what she intended with the Senior Lecturer in Health Studies responsible for health visiting courses in the institution where she worked as a lecturer. The S/L gave her the names of the Nurse Managers in charge of health visiting in the three health districts for which training in health visiting was provided by the institution. She wrote to each of these, enclosing a copy of her research proposal and asking if they would be willing to give her access to the health visitors working under them. Each of them wrote back and suggested that she went to see them; she did so, and each agreed to her request. In each district the Nurse Manager provided her with the names and telephone numbers of health visitors working in different settings (rural, urban, working-class or middle-class areas) and with greater or less professional experience. She contacted selected ones and explained what she wanted, and all agreed to participate.

She carried out interviews with health visitors at their place of work. Each interview lasted between 1 and 1½ hours. Beforehand, she prepared a list of topic areas she wanted to cover, to act as an aide memoire, but the basic approach was 'life-history' interviewing: she started by asking each informant why she had decided to train as a health visitor, and from this got them talking generally about their work and their professional careers. After each of the interviews she went out with each health visitor for a half or a whole day, observing what they did with 'cases' and talking to them further. This was to give her a greater familiarity with what health visitors actually do and an opportunity to chart their day-to-day work.

This research was very much centred on health visitors' conceptions of their own roles. If the researcher had been more interested in organizational constraints and/or official goals, she would have interviewed more senior staff. If the focus had been organization at the local level, a better approach might have been to concentrate on certain 'patches' and try to interview doctors, practice nurses, midwives, etc., as well as health visitors (and perhaps social workers – particularly if she had wanted to explore questions of the mistreatment of children). With a focus on whether health visitors deliver what their clients want, interviews with the clients themselves would have been indispensable.

12

Analysing text

This chapter is concerned mostly with the analysis of qualitative data: filed notes from participant observation, notes on qualitative interviews, audio-tapes or secondary textual sources – diaries, newspapers, articles, historical documents and so on. All of these may be seen in some sense as 'text' – verbal material not structured for the purposes of the research as is the output of a survey or an experiment, but awaiting such structure as you can impose on it or draw out of it. Qualitative data, even more than quantitative, do not speak for themselves, however much they may appear to do so; they need to be analysed. (Text may also be analysed by quantitative methods – measuring the frequency of occurrence of a topic or a concept or a word, or the space given to it in a report, or in some other way reducing the complexity of the material to analysable numbers. Here the methods discussed in Chapters 8–11 would apply.) In this chapter we shall talk about the descriptive use of qualitative materials, about holistic analysis in terms of 'cases', and about analyses in terms of the detailed content of interviews or documents. These forms of analysis blur into each other, as we shall see, but it is useful to separate them out and consider them separately here.

The first step is to get the material into a form in which it can be ordered and analysed. Tapes need to be transcribed, for example – or if you do not have the time for this (an hour's interview takes several hours to transcribe) then you at least need to take detailed notes from the tapes, plus an 'index' of what is where (by noting the counter reading on your tape recorder which corresponds with each topic). You will need to work out a system for locating material – perhaps case numbers or day records, page numbers within them, and line numbers within the pages – so that it is possible to locate particular references easily at a later stage. You will need to read all the material you have collected, to familiarize yourself fully with it and form a tentative overall impression of it. You need also to establish a filing system. This may be physical: storing relevant material together in one place, such as a series of clearly labelled envelopes or wallet files. In this case you will need multiple copies of all your material, as some of it may well need to be stored under a number of different headings. Alternatively, your filing system may be indexical – you may 'store' references in the form of location indicators, on file-cards or on the computer. (Indexical 'storage' is easier in the early stages, involving less physical transfer of material, but physical means of storage are far less trouble when it comes time to write up, as you have your source material already segmented and organized into 'sets'.)

The amount of data that you will have collected may well be vast, and you may feel that it is a daunting task that faces you. The first thing to do is to focus down and remind yourself what the *purpose* of your inquiry was, what you were interested in finding out. You will then realize that quite a lot of the material you have collected is not relevant to this. It may be interesting in its own right, and you may want to keep it to analyse at some time in the future, but it is not needed for your immediate purposes. When we interviewed mothers whose children had learning difficulties, for example, one copy of the transcribed interviews filled six or eight box-files. A relatively small amount of that was relevant to what we were originally investigating: the load on the mother as compared with mothers of 'unlabelled' children, and the social and self-stigmatizing that occurred (Abbott and Sapsford 1987b, among other reports). More detailed material from a few particularly interesting 'cases' yielded another paper, on the *diversity* of mothers' experiences (Abbott and Sapsford 1986). The rest sits in the cupboard, brought out only for teaching examples, until such time as one of us wants to use it for another purpose – perhaps some kind of analysis of socialization and growing up, as we elicited the women's life histories as well as their current circumstances.

Qualitative description

Much of your material will be descriptive – describing situations and events – and you will want to use it in writing a descriptive account in your final report. Description could be a main purpose of your research. For example, in some research on evaluating Enterprise in Higher Education which one of us (Abbott) is doing, the report on qualitative evaluation of individual enterprise programmes requires that there be a description of the programme, including the aims and objectives of its leaders, what they did and what the outcomes were. The descriptive material may itself begin the analysis by the way it is ordered under headings – e.g. in the EHE example, the programme as a whole and individual programmes as broad headings, and relevant sub-headings within each broad category. (You will find that much of the work of qualitative analysis involves sorting into hierarchical categories, in one way or another.) Careful reading of your data and thinking about what 'story' your report is to tell will enable you to decide on relevant sub-headings. All of the material for the descriptive account can be collected together and put in a file or series of envelopes labelled 'descriptive material'.

Under some circumstances it may be relevant to work through each case or setting or visit or whatever in some detail, organizing the material under relevant sub-headings. For example, if you had life-history data on a person, you could separate the purely descriptive material from the rest and organize it chronologically and under separate headings – e.g. 'childhood relations with parents', 'education' . . . Even where this is not a relevant way of proceeding, however, it is good practice to write brief notes 'telling the story' of each case – summarizing in a few sentences what the informant has to say about himself or herself, his or her life and the topics which are of particular interest to you, or what the significance of the setting or programme appeared to be to you and to the participants. (This may also allow your reflexive notes about particular data-collection sessions to have some impact on the analysis.) You may never use these overall summary accounts in your written report, but they will help to shape your analysis, and comparing them across cases may allow interesting patterns to emerge. They are also a good early point of the analysis at which to think about the informant as a whole person. (Note, however, that a proportion of published research on medicine, psychotherapy, counselling and social work draws on this kind of impressionistic material – 'case notes' – as a prime source, treating it as factual rather than as field-notes of a process of participant observation and failing to acknowledge the role of the researcher/practitioner in the construction of the data.)

Case analysis

Qualitative analysis which goes beyond description consists essentially of the processes of sorting, comparing/contrasting and consolidating. Most of what follows involves, in one way or another, sorting cases or propositions or utterances or words into categories such that the members resemble each other and differ from other categories in ways which are of interest to the researcher.

The simplest form of such analysis is 'impressionistic' case analysis – sorting cases into 'heaps' which have something in common which they do not share with other cases. This is what we did at one stage of the analysis of the interviews with mothers of children with learning difficulties. We read through the transcripts of interviews and formed impressions about the mothers who were speaking, holistically rather than on the basis of any particular detailed feature of what was said. On this basis we sorted mothers (families) into those who effectively denied that a problem existed, those who acknowledged that a problem existed and were trying to cope with it (distinguishing between those who had some expressed long-term strategy and those who appeared to be keeping their heads above water on a more day-to-day basis), and those who had managed to reconstrue the situation as one with positive advantages. This kind of analysis is faithful to the data in the sense that it draws on the interview material and uses it as a basis for classification. It is obviously also open, however, to being very strongly influenced by the researchers' previous ideas, because there are no rigourous criteria for determining what the criteria shall be, other than the impressions of the researchers.

More rigorous analysis involves more detailed examination of categories within interviews, rather than just comparison between cases, as we shall see. Even so, however, you ought to return to the holistic consideration of cases at some point of the analysis. In writing up your analysis you will want to give more detailed accounts of a subset of cases – possibly to illustrate different categories or types that you have 'discovered' in your research. For example, in the EHE research the final report could include a detailed analysis of a small number of programmes as examples illustrating the range of programmes and the kinds of enterprise they represent. Alternatively, the cases could be selected to illustrate successful and unsuccessful programmes or to illustrate the types of problems encountered by programme leaders in implementing the programmes, and/or students, and/or collaborating employers. All the material relevant to each of the cases needs to be collected together – one file or envelope per case or one index entry.

Content analysis

In your subsequent analysis and write-up of these cases you would look for similarities and differences between them. This is the main process of bringing order to the material, organizing it into patterns, categories and descriptive units. It is now possible to purchase computer programmes that can assist in the content analysis of qualitative data, but most of us still have to do some or all of it 'by hand'. Content analysis needs to be done on all the data, including material which you have already sorted out to use for description or as illustrative cases.

The first step is to look for all concepts and make an index of them. A computer qualitative analysis programme will do this for you, as indeed will some word-processing packages. Using such a programme, you would need to look at its output, eliminate the vary rare concepts (after looking to see where they occurred, in case they were important) and grouping others together because they clearly expressed similar ideas even if different words were used. If you have to do it by hand you need to re-read every bit of the data, noting down all the categories that are relevant to the purpose of your analysis – and probably some that do not seem relevant at present, but might seem so at a later stage. First you would look across the paragraphs to see what overall topic areas came up – work, home, geographical area and its significance, the children and so on. Each of these may want breaking down further: children's health, the children's school as a place, the children's school performance as a measure of their worth, sports activities and so on. Finally, you might still want or need to do a full textual analysis, looking for every descriptive category the informant uses (in which case you might seriously consider whether you can get hold of computer assistance).

As a brief example of this kind of content analysis, consider the following short extract from one of our interviews with a mother whose child had learning difficulties:

RJS: What was Wyvern like when you first came here?

Mrs Weaver: It's built up a lot since we first came here. It used to be very, very quiet, very quiet.

RJS: Did you have this house then?

Mrs Weaver: No we lived in Dunstone Estate when we first moved here . . . and then we moved up here. A very friendly place, I think, Wyvern . . . It's nice. And everybody's accepted Carl [mentally handicapped son], that's what we like. In a normal way.

In this brief extract we can see a number of 'place' references qualified by adjectives – 'quiet' (as a term of approval), 'friendly', 'nice'. The topic of the mentally handicapped son has also come up, leading to concepts of 'accepting' (by people around) and 'in a *normal* way'. Another person might characterize the same place as 'quiet' (in a pejorative sense), 'nosy', 'dull'. Contrasting people who look at it in the one light or the other, we might find other differences between them – in demographic characteristics, or in the way they see their mentally handicapped children as fitting into the life of the area – and we would be on the way towards model-building. Analysis proceeds by constantly comparing and contrasting interview scripts, looking for similarities and differences, and trying to find which characteristics seem to vary systematically together.

Note that there are two levels at which this kind of analysis can be carried out. On the one hand, you can categorize the material in terms of your own previous interests. In the EHE example, for instance, the categories which are likely to emerge are very likely to be conditioned by the focus of the research. If your enquiry had a wider and less directed focus – e.g. 'What is it like being a prisoner, or a patient or a mother' – then you would want to start further back, by trying to list *all* the descriptive nouns, adjectives and phrases that look even vaguely relevant to the enquiry, clustering them by similarity, and looking further at ones that are at all common or appear to express strong feeling, *before* focusing on particular questions that may be of concern to the researcher. Except where the focus of the research is very narrow and/or the interviews were very directive, the latter is probably a better procedure than the former.

When you have a list of categories you can group them into sets of similar relevance and begin to map their relationships. For example, in our research into community care for children with special learning difficulties we grouped all the concepts relating to 'husband', 'children', 'mother', 'other kin', the ones relating to 'neighbours', to 'schools' and so on. These were clusters which appeared to make sense to the informants and which made sense to us. There is no 'magic formula' for how concepts are to be clustered – you are just looking for ones that appear to 'go together', express the same underlying idea or are related to the same topic sub-area. The clusters can again be grouped more broadly in further analysis – 'husband' and 'children' go together as 'nuclear family', 'mother' and 'other kin' go together as kin network. At this stage, as far as is possible, the themes and categories should come from the data rather than from previous ideas – they should reflect patterns found more than patterns looked for.

Meta-analysis

The aim so far has been to try to characterize the informants' worlds in the terms in which they themselves see them. The next step – what one might call 'second-order analysis' – is to go beyond the informants' concepts and start trying to build theory at another level. Patterns may suggest themselves in the data. For example, the people who saw places such as Wyvern as 'nice' may tend to be those with mentally handicapped children of school age or preschool children who were not handicapped; those who saw it as 'dull' might have older children, or very young children who were handicapped. We hasten to say that this is *not* the pattern we found in our interview study. If it *had* occurred, however, we might have speculated about the different needs of the four types of families, for activities for themselves and the children, and started building a model of the school-age mentally handicapped child as having some of the social function of the preschool non-handicapped child (i.e. constituting the same kind of burden). We might look for further confirmation in what informants did *not* say. Might it be the case, for example, that those who found Wyvern dull talked about a need for entertainment or relaxation, while those who found it 'nice' did not. Was this a difference which held up across time – were the latter less likely to mention entertainment and relaxation even when talking about their lives before marriage? Or might it be an adaptation to circumstances: did the latter fail to mention relatives or friends able to look after the child while they went out? Or might it be the perception of the former which was at fault: might it be they who lacked a support network and, therefore, felt confined, while the latter were, in fact, able to get out when they wanted to? All of this is going substantially beyond what any one informant might want to say about his or her life, but it is still analysis grounded in data, and the informants might still recognize themselves in this account.

This is a particular example of a general principle – looking for how respondents typify, or stereotype or categorize the field of the research, and drawing generalized conclusions from the patterns that emerge. In the example above we were looking at judgements of place, but it might have been judgements they make and express about other people, or government agencies, or medical procedures, depending on the topic area of the research. For example, research on nurses has shown them typifying patients into 'good' and 'bad' categories, and the category within which a patient was placed has an effect on the ways in which the nurses treated and interacted with him or her. In our research on mothers, they typified health visitors as 'helpful' and 'unhelpful', and separately into 'informed', 'ignorant' and 'bossy' ('ignorant, but not prepared to admit it'). Relatives were categorized as 'helpful', unhelpful' or 'indifferent'. The categories were not necessarily related; a health visitor could be ignorant, but helpful. Sometimes a typificatory scheme will be used by all respondents. Sometimes it will be used by some, with others using a different one; in the research above, for example, some mothers regarded *all* health visitors (and, we thought, all *conceivable* health visitors) as 'unhelpful'. Sometimes it will be unique to a particular informant. Once the typologies have been identified and the material to do with them sorted out, it is possible to start asking serious questions about the content: what is it that is seen as making 'a good patient', 'a helpful health visitor', 'an indifferent relative'.

Exercise 32: Analysis of interview data

Try your hand at some analysis, with the following brief extract from one of our interviews with mothers of mentally handicapped children. Our initial shot at it is given at the end of the chapter. (All names are fictitious. The phrases in square brackets are our interpolations.)

> RJS: You think Kings School [school for ESN(S) children] has been bringing him on?
>
> Mrs Weaver: Oh yeah, marvellous, yeah! He's only been there twelve months, and we've noticed a vast, er, change in him . . .
> . . . it was me, I pushed, I didn't want him to go to Kings because I'd heard so much of, I'm a bit frightened of that sort of thing, I, I don't like illness, you know?
>
> RJS: Hm.
>
> Mrs Weaver: And I'd heard so much about all the terrible sort of cases there . . . But [the ESN(M) school] wasn't really the sort of place for him. It's for maladjusted rather than handicapped children, you know. And I mean, they did all they could for him, but the last twelve, eighteen months he was there he was ever so miserable . . . they're very good at Kings, you know. I mean, if there's any problems they're straight away, sort of, on to you, telling you. They involve you in everything. And as I say, he's happy there.
>
> RJS: Does he get, does he get on with the other children?
>
> Mrs Weaver: Yeah, yeah, he does, everyone seems to like him. But Carl's like that, he's got a way with him, everybody sort of takes to him . . .
>
> PAA: What, he went to a, to a nursery, did he, at [the ESN(M) school]?
>
> Mrs Weaver: Yes, he started when he was, I think he was, I can't really remember how old he was, he must have been about three, and he went there until last year, as I say.
>
> PAA: Then he was assessed as educable?
>
> Mrs Weaver: Oh, yeah . . . The last time he was assessed there, it was Mr Bowen, the what do you call it?
>
> PAA: Psychologist.
>
> Mrs Weaver: Yeah, that's right. He said 'Oh, he's not yet reached the mental

age of a two-year-old' and I was most insulted, you know. I mean, I know
he has, I mean, a two-year-old didn't do what Carl was doing.

RJS: Yes

Mrs Weaver: Um, and I think it's unfair that they assess them like they do. I
mean he, he took Carl into a room, and Carl had never seen him before,
and he wouldn't do anything for him, and he kept saying 'He doesn't know
where his nose is, doesn't know where this, that and the other is', and I felt
like saying, 'Well, you get him in here, and I'll show you whether he knows
where it is', you know.

RJS: Yes [laugh]

Mrs Weaver: I mean, he'd not even seen the man before. Carl was very afraid
of strangers then . . . But this psychologist, I mean I don't really think he
gave him the benefit of the doubt then. I mean, I knew that Carl knew them
things, but I'm not the sort of person to say 'Well, I know that he knows
that', you know.

(Working with textual material *as* text, some research will call for a leap
straight into a form of meta-analysis. Sometimes the interest focuses not on
the detailed content, but on what is expressed by it – ideologies, discourses,
settled 'worked-views' which emerge from the way that topics are discussed.
This is sometimes called 'critical analysis'. It has most often been applied
in the analysis of government documents and the utterances of politicians,
particularly in the criminological field, looking for politically informed views
of the world that are implicit in what is being said and taken for granted,
unanalysed, by the speaker or writer. Similar work has been done by
feminists on texts about education, family and social policy. Such work is
necessarily impressionistic, but what emerges can be very illuminating.)

A final stage in the analysis is to go beyond the patterns that are emergent
in the data themselves and try to *explain* them – a theoretical interpretation.
In our research on the mothers, for example, we typified them on the basis of
our analysis of the material we had collected. We also put their experiences
into the context of policies of community care and examined the extent to
which our findings 'matched' those of other researchers. Furthermore, we
tried to locate them (in the first half of the book, which you were not directed
to read) within a set of historical processes which makes sense at the same
time of their reactions to their own circumstances, the reactions of others to
the visibly handicapped children, and the nature and development of government policy in this area.

However far you go along the road of analysis, meta-analysis and theoretical interpretation – even if you do not get far beyond 'description' – it
is important to 'test' tentative conclusions by looking back through the
material for contradictory evidence – for material that will challenge or
question the interpretation you have put on your findings. It is also
important to be continually reflexive – to consider how your purpose, your
training, your reading, your background assumptions and your prejudices
have influenced both the collection of the data and your analysis of them. It

can be useful to write notes relevant to this as you are doing the analysis, and it is certainly wise to try to keep a log or diary of the stages of the analysis. These themselves become data for analysis. A good starting point is to write down all your initial ideas, past findings, hopes for the research, ideas about what you think you might find, at the outset of the research, and continue to make notes as you go along.

Further reading

Burgess, Robert (1984). *In the Field*. London: Allen and Unwin.
Hammersley, Martyn and Atkinson, Paul (1989). *Ethnography: Principles in Practice*. London: Routledge.
Hyener, R.H. (1985). 'Some guidelines for the phenomenological analysis of interview data' *Human Problems*, 8, 279–303.
Patton, Michael (1987). *How to Use Qualitative Methods in Evaluation*. Beverly Hills: Sage.
Plummer, Kenneth (1983). *Documents of Life*. London: Allen and Unwin.

Specimen answer to Exercise 32

The overall story is a clear one, of assessment by an educational psychologist whom Mrs Weaver sees as incompetent, testing her child under conditions where he could not possibly do his best. This is what she was telling us in this passage. It is not clear from what is here whether this is seen as a failure of this particular psychologist or as characteristic of the breed.

The passage is a brief one, but descriptive categories do emerge which would be worth following up through the rest of the script and other scripts:

1 Describing herself, Mrs Weaver talks about herself with negative emotion as 'pushing' on a particular occasion and as 'frightened of that sort of thing' [ESN(S) cases], and in positive terms as 'not the sort of person to' push her views forward. Carl, positively, is described as 'everyone seems to like him . . . he's got a way with him'. 'Afraid of strangers', applied to Carl, does not seem to be a negative label so much as a neutral description of a childhood stage. This begins to give us a basis for understanding her ways of categorizing other people, which could be followed up in the rest of the interview and contrasted with other interviews.

2 The description of the assessment process is interestingly juridical, in the use of the phrase 'didn't give him the benefit of the doubt' and in the repeated description of it as 'unfair'.

3 We should note that, like any other parent, Mrs Weaver's honour is bound up in the outcome of the test: 'He said "Oh, he's not yet reached the mental age of a two-year-old", and I was most insulted.'

4 The terms used to describe children who have been classified as mentally handicapped are interesting: 'that sort of thing, I don't like illness', 'terrible sort of cases there', 'maladjusted' (of the 'mild' children), 'handicapped' of her own (without the qualifying 'mentally').

5 What is missing, from this passage and, in fact, from the whole interview, is any use of phrases such as 'these children' to refer to mentally handicapped children as a class. Mrs Weaver does not show the signs evident in some of the interviews of classing them together as something different from herself. On the contrary, the force of her early remarks about fears of Kings School on the one hand, and the description of children in the other school as not really handicapped, is to separate him from both and render him unique.

13

Participant observation and self-evaluation

Much of this book has been about the evaluation of practice on one form or another; one of our major themes has been that there is not just one kind of evaluation research, but many different ways. In this chapter we look at the broadest, most naturalistic and least prestructured form of research: observing in a natural setting, as a participant. This is one way in which situations have been explored from the perspective of the participants with (ideally) minimal imposition of researchers' or managements' preconceived ideas. It is also one form in which your own practice may be investigated in the widest possible way, looking not at how some particular practice works, but at how, in general, your professional life is lived, what it means and what the implicit 'working rules' are.

Deliberately, we have not set practical exercises in this chapter. Participant observation might be seen as the most dangerous way in which research can be conducted. It can be destructive of relationships, it can upset and side-track your professional practice, and the 'methodological imagination' can sometimes be stretched to the point where your very sense of identity comes under attack. You can also do great damage to the people in the context you are researching, if the practice of your research is not constantly monitored by you and by others. It is not a form of research to be undertaken without supervision from someone who has been 'in the field' and knows the problems, and from an academic base where, at frequent intervals, you can change roles and discharge the tensions and self-doubts which have accumulated during the fieldwork.

Covert participant observation

In this section we shall talk about classic participant observation, where a researcher becomes part of a context without participants knowing that he or she is a researcher – *covert* (hidden, secret) participant observation. A first and substantial problem, clearly, is how the researcher is to become part of the context. Sometimes it is possible to join by legitimate means: one may do participant observation in a hospital by coming in legitimately as a patient, for example, or by becoming a student nurse, or by taking a job as a hospital porter, or by joining the 'Friends of the Hospital' and acquiring the role of the person who takes a trolley of books round or the person who works in the hospital shop. If you wanted to do research on child-care and you had children, it would be easy enough to join the relevant playgroup or parent–teacher association or to place your children with child-minders and take notes of what goes on. In many contexts it is not possible to *join* in this way, however. If you wanted to do research on student doctors, for example, it might not be possible for you to join as a medical student. It might be possible, however, for you to pass yourself off as a student doctor – to dress similarly and to attend the same lectures and demonstrations. Research on youths, on unemployed persons, on 'deviant' sexual groups and on religious sects has been carried out by this stratagem of *passing* – pretending to be a relevant person within the context.

A second problem is data-collection, because quite clearly any sign that you were taking notes as you went along would destroy your credibility as a genuine participant. Sometimes it is possible to take notes in a covert manner, but within the normal actions of a participant – if paper-work is normally conducted, or if one can seem to be reading something and scribbling in the margins. More often it is necessary to leave the scene from time to time to take notes (going to the toilet, for example – the first sign of a covert participant observer is often an apparently weak bladder!), or 'writing up' at the end of a session or the end of the day. Whatever stratagem has to be adopted, it is crucial to make as full a record as possible, as soon as possible, before events and occurrences have begun to be re-arranged in memory.

The full-blown participant enquiry is not just an intuitive description. At first one goes into the field in a descriptive way, establishes a role, learns the part and just tries to get a feel for what is going on. As the observation progresses, however, ideas will begin to emerge as to what it is important to say about the context, and progressively one will begin to pay more attention to some features of the situation than to others. This *progressive focusing* is the first stage of theory-building – trying to establish what is important or interesting in the situation. As time goes on the theme will become clearer and a tentative theoretical model of the situation will begin to be put forward. This will be refined and tested by:

1 *Theoretical sampling*: testing the generality and the boundaries of an idea. One might look initially for very similar situations or aspects of the one situation, to show that the model had some generality. Next one might look for very dissimilar contexts, to establish the boundaries of the ideas. Finally, one might systematically sample groups who were like the original one in every respect but one, to test particular hypotheses. For example, working in a hospital on nurses, you would check that your

emerging ideas held for the night shift as well as for the day nurses, for all types of wards, for auxiliaries, aids and students, as well as for qualified nurses. You might then try to see whether they held for sisters, for doctors, for the hospital management or whether they were confined to the 'shop floor' of the caring staff, and you might look at patients and their relatives to see whether they had generality beyond the caring staff. Finally, you might start making very specific comparisons – male nurses and female ones, older nurses and younger ones, theatre nurses and ward nurses – according to what your emerging model predicted might be of interest.

2 *Analytic induction*: given a model which seems to be well delineated after this kind of process, a final stage is to test it against 'unlikely cases'. You deliberately look for cases which falsify your picture or do not seem to fit the model, and to the extent that they cannot be 'explained away' you try to re-formulate the model to take account of them. This process goes on until you are very sure of the boundaries of what you want to say and no new information appears to be emerging – the point of *theoretical saturation*.

(We should perhaps point out that very few projects get as far as this; what we are describing is an ideal and complete project, probably representing several years' work.)

A problem with all participant work, but particularly acute in covert participant observation, is the marginal nature of the researcher. Marginality is essential, so that the natural situation shall not be changed by the researcher's presence and so that he or she can stand back from the taken-for-granted nature of the situation, and see it in a more complete and analytic way even than the participants. Marginality is very difficult to maintain, however. If the researcher remains uninvolved in the situation, the value of being a participant is lost. (It is also a very lonely and disorienting experience.) If he or she 'goes native' and becomes a true participant to the extent that the researcher's detachment is lost, then the research suffers. Finding a place between these two extremes which is effective and comfortable is very difficult. Wherever the researcher is located, short of going completely native, anxiety and stress will follow, as the researcher tries to balance the two roles while 'maintaining cover', concealing the research role and acting plausibly as what he or she purports to be in the situation.

Covert participant observation incurs further costs, in personal and ethical terms. To the extent that the researcher manages to maintain cover, he or she may be drawn into disturbing the situation by the very role that is being played: researchers have found themselves almost becoming gang-leaders, for instance, because they know more about the police than the average youth and their advice is therefore good. They may also find themselves dragged into behaviour which is normal for participants (and they will 'blow their cover' if they abstain), but which they may not wish to undertake. People researching in shops and offices have had to condone pilfering, for example, or been invited to take part, and research on youth may drag the researcher into vandalism or violence. At the other extreme, if the researcher fails to maintain cover, he or she will be exposed as a fraud who had been building up relationships for the sake of research; at the least this will hurt, dismay or anger the true participants, and they may take steps against him or her as a consequence. Perhaps the worst problem, however, is how to live with the fact of building relationships and enjoying confidences with the intention of using them for a purpose other than that of the participants. The researcher may be able to cope with this if the consequences of the research are seen as important (research into commercial malpractice and the 'crimes of the powerful', for instance) or if the research is seen as putting the participants' point of view to the world, but it remains, nonetheless, an uncomfortable position. Many social scientists would now argue that covert participant observation is always ethically unacceptable.

Exercise 33: Advantages and disadvantages of overt observation

Spend a few minutes thinking about observation in which the researcher's identity as researcher is *not* concealed. What advantages do you see, and what would be the disadvantages, as compared with covert participant observation?

Overt observation

Much participant research is carried out quite openly, with the researcher being readily identifiable as a researcher. (See, for example, the Kirkham paper which we looked at in Chapter 4). Declaring what you are saves many of the ethical qualms of covert work – no-one is deceived and participants know that you cannot necessarily be expected to 'go along with' everything that they do. You also have a freedom to 'move around in the field' which is often denied the covert observer. For example, one group of covert observers had themselves admitted as patients to a mental hospital (Caudill *et al.* 1952), and learned a great deal about how patients are treated and how they treat each other. Being labelled as patients, however, they could not also observe the nurses or the doctors on their own ground and socialize with them as equals. If they had been openly researching, it would have been quite natural for them (indeed, probably required of them), to talk to people at all levels and to make themselves available in a wide range of circumstances. You are also freer to ask questions. As the 'amiable incompetent' in a covert role you can pretend to be a little stupid or ignorant in order to elicit material, but the extent to which you can do so without 'blowing your cover' is strictly limited. As a researcher no-one necessarily expects you to understand what is going on, so you are free to ask.

The disadvantage is the risk of *reactivity*: that your presence and the way you behave is altering the situation and that things would be quite different if you were not there. This is a risk even in covert work – by taking a role you necessarily affect the situation. In overt work you have to make substantial allowances for the fact that people know they are being researched – something akin to a Hawthorne Effect – and for the fact that they are undoubtedly trying to 'sell you a line' of one sort or another. As time goes on and people become used to your presence you may feel that this tendency is diminishing, but you can never be sure. You may also not necessarily feel that all the ethical problems of covert work are overcome; it is still the case that you are building relationships for your own particular purposes, to gain data rather than just to relate.

Another problem even with 'open' participant research is encountered where any kind of 'power relationship' is involved – where the setting in which the research is being carried out involves clients or patients or pupils or inmates. Not infrequently when researchers say that they were open participants in a setting they mean that their identity was known to the professionals in it – the doctors, nurses, social workers, health visitors, teachers, prison staff. Rather less often is their presence as researchers explained or even made obvious to the patients, clients, pupils or inmates. Intimate or private aspects of clients' or pupils' lives may be reported in research which did not ask their consent to this. It is not entirely clear, in all situations, whether asking consent would be in the patients' interests: it could distort the relationship with the professionals and interfere with the effectiveness of the service they require, if they were aware that they were under research scrutiny. However, whether participant research is ethical under such circumstances must therefore be a matter for debate. Furthermore, even where consent is given by clients or pupils or patients, it is not clear how free that consent is: where someone requires a service from a professional (as in health care) or is under a professional's authority (as in schools), it is difficult to refuse such requests.

Another problem with overt participation (and, indeed, with 'open' interviewing) is that the informants may not have realized the 'rules of the game' as seen by the researcher. In interviews, the informant is well aware that what is said to the tape recorder will be used for the research. He or she may *not* be aware that what is said 'off-stage' during coffee-breaks or casual meetings will also be used. (The researcher may agree not to use material which is declared to be 'not for the tape recorder', but there is no way that he or she can *avoid* using it; it is *there*, in the researcher's mind, during the analysis, and it must necessarily shape how the formally recorded material is interpreted.) Similarly, a teacher may quite happily allow a researcher to participate in classroom sessions. He or she may not feel, however, that the contract stretches to the (inevitable) use of remarks and conversations overheard in the staff-room or even the toilets.

The overarching methodological problem with reports based on participant observation data, whether covert or overt, is the problem of validity: why anyone should take your word that what you claim to have seen and heard is what any other reasonable person would have extracted from the situation. Inevitably, however much you illustrate your report with quotations and extracts from field-notes, the reader has to trust you to have interpreted what you saw, heard and experienced in the same way that he or she would have interpreted it. The two guarantors of validity to which you may make appeal are *triangulation* and *reflexivity*. Triangulation, a metaphor drawn from navigation, means taking more than one bearing on a point in order to locate it uniquely. In research terms it means being able to show that more than one source has been used, each with its own bias, but not necessarily the same in each case. Thus, observation is supplemented with interviews, to show that what you conclude from observing behaviour is what the participants also understand by it, or at least that what you conclude makes sense to the participants. One may draw on informal conversations overheard in staff-rooms, toilets, etc. to supplement formal interviews. One may look for diaries, letters, articles which participants have written for the newspapers, etc., in order to extend the range of perspectives. Ideally, one may have more than one observer, perhaps located in different parts of the 'research field', to elicit different viewpoints and different interpretations. Each of these sources leads to an account, and no account is necessarily privileged over other accounts, but to the extent that differently based accounts appear to agree we may have more faith in the result. To the extent that they do not agree, further research may be needed before you are in a position to report.

Reflexivity is of even more importance. At every stage of the research, right from the initial introductions, you must be thinking about how the participants are making sense of you and your presence, what you are taking for granted or learning as new about them, and how what you are doing may be shaping particular pieces of data or the whole relationship between you and participants. This is important for three reasons. It acts as a form of self-monitoring, so that you can spot something 'going wrong' and be at pains to correct it. It is, itself, a form of data analysis, one way in which you find your way through the morass of material towards the underlying model which simplifies and makes sense of what is going on. Finally, it is the basis of your self-justification in the eventual report, your way of showing that others should believe that your interpretations are reasonable ones.

Observation in the workplace

There are obvious advantages in being a 'participant observer' in your own workplace, but equally obvious disadvantages, given what we have said above. The major advantage is that you already have a natural role, the one you are carrying out in your job. There is no question of 'joining' or 'passing': you are already *in*. Equally important, at a practical level, you have no need to find your way through a maze of 'gatekeepers': you are already in the situation and can take whatever notes it pleases you to take with no need for anyone's permission. (You may find your superiors feel they should have been consulted if you ever decide to publish anything from your notes, but if what is at stake is a piece of 'internal research', examining and drawing conclusions from the practice and ethos of your unit, then no one can restrain you from doing it.) The overwhelming problem, however, is that you *are* a part of what you are examining. It is very difficult indeed to stand back from your normal practices and see them as anything other than the only or best way of coping with the situation. It is very difficult to stand back from the normal assumptions and typifications of your trade, and see them as anything other than inevitable and sensible. (Sensible they may be, but it is a necessary part of taking the research stance that you do not regard them as inevitable, but try to see them as what *happens* to be there, among the wide range of what *might* have been there.) All this may require you to put aside your own values and goals and your professional socialization; you work in a situation with which you may have struggled for years to make it familiar, but the research requires that you stand back from it and make it strange to yourself. Most difficult of all is to put down your own automatic assumptions about what is normal, sensible, right in any given situation and ask yourself, first, whether others hold the same values and, secondly, whether what you all do may also (or instead) serve some other purpose.

A good starting-point for such research is autobiography. Spend a good period of time trying to describe your own life and values on paper, from before you ever joined the given line of work to the present day, covering what you think the job is for, what you want out of it (not necessarily the same question), where you would like to go next, what you think brings others into the job, what you think motivates them, whether it motivates you. Study this record as if it were a set of life history interviews conducted with someone else, and analyse it for major themes; learn from these themes what your own preconceptions are likely to be. Better still – because diary-writing of this kind is still shaped by the presence of an 'other in the head', an other who looks for socially acceptable positions – get someone else to interview you and ask the questions; others can push you to clarify ideas which might seem to you self-evidently clear when you write them down. Best of all, do both – but writing the autobiography before undergoing the interview, because both are fallible accounts and the power of an interviewer to make you clarify what you might otherwise have passed over is likely to affect any subsequent account that you write.

Whether working covertly or overtly, you have to be very careful about your working relationships when researching your own work setting. A clear distinction must be made here between 'research' – activities leading to a publication or a report to management or even a set of conclusions announced in public – and that monitoring of your own daily practice, and the practice of staff for whom you are responsible, which is a necessary part of most professional jobs and can benefit from the application of research techniques and the research imagination. The latter must be done and, therefore, should be done well. The former is something undertaken additionally, and it faces the ethical problems of participant research which have been discussed earlier in the chapter – problems of interfering in the working lives of colleagues and clients/patients, with or without their consent. You will necessarily find yourself asking questions which probe into a level of intimacy which may not be appropriate for the stage of acquaintanceship which you have reached. Even if you do not find people 'cooling' to your inquisitiveness, you will find yourself in possession of information which would normally be appropriate to a much closer level of intimacy than you have so far reached, because you will have paid attention to people in a way that you would not normally as part of your everyday working life. Handling this at the personal level can be a problem. In open research – or even more, in covert research when your cover is blown and people realize that you are taking notes on them – you can become labelled as a spy or a reporter, someone with whom interaction has to be very guarded.

Perhaps more difficult still is the effect of researching your own working *milieu* and its 'normal rules' on your relationship to your own professional practice. Our professional lives depend in large part on the values which we have incorporated, and on a set of working practices and priorities which have become largely unconscious by the time that we have become competent at our trades. To stand back and question these can be like the priest questioning his faith and his commitment to the church – once we 'make the familiar strange', it may *remain* strange, and we may not be able to find our way back to professional commitment. The methodological imagination involves a great degree of self-questioning, and those (which is most of us) who are unsure of themselves should be careful how deeply they question something as crucial to their public and private identities as their professional roles and practices.

A way round some of these problems is the kind of collaborative approach we shall discuss in Chapter 14. If a whole group of you get together to assess and evaluate how you do your job together, then the loneliness is dispelled, you are not faced with taking the role of the spy, and there are others with whom you can talk out personal problems that may arise in the course of the research. Three warnings, however:

1 There is no 'natural situation' for you to explore: what you have is the contrived situation of a group of people who are all committed to a programme of research and improvement, and who are all watching themselves and each other. The 'autobiography' stage, or prior interviewing of each other, is particularly important here.
2 A Hawthorne Effect, or something akin, is inevitable: what you will be exploring is not normal practice, but how practice can be improved by and during collaborative evaluation.
3 Once started, such an undertaking is difficult to stop, and the atmosphere of the unit can become very intense and critical.

Further reading

Burgess, Robert (1984). *In the Field*. London: Allen and Unwin.
Hammersley, Martyn and Atkinson, Paul (1989). *Ethnography: Principles in Practice*. London: Routledge.
Patton, Michael (1987). *How to Use Qualitative Methods in Evaluation*. Beverly Hills; Sage.
Taylor, S.J. and Bogden, R. (1984). *An Introduction to Qualitative Research Methods*. Chichester; Wiley.
For a straightforward account of a piece of participant work, see:
Cavendish, Ruth (1982). *Women on the Line*. London: Routledge and Kegan Paul.

14

Evaluation of single cases

In a sense, all research is about single cases. However we proceed, we collect measurements, responses or accounts from informants one at a time, or observe contexts one at a time. Generally, we aim to cover a fair number of single cases and in some sense add the results together – literally in the case of quantitative research, and in the sense of pitting one case against another in qualitative research. We build up the numbers to eliminate or deal with the idiosyncratic variation which is inherent in the single case, or – putting it another way – to overcome sampling error and establish typicality or representativeness. We use comparison or control groups to explore the boundaries of our conclusions and establish their validity. Even in 'open' research (open interviewing, participant observation) we go for substantial numbers and use comparison groups where this is feasible (see, for example, the Abbott and Sapsford (1987b) paper which we discussed in Chapter 3). Much research into practice in the areas of health and social work, however, necessarily consists of single-case evaluation, seeing what treatment works for the particular patient or client. In this chapter we look at what can be done with single cases.

Virtually all single-case research is either purely descriptive or focused on the evaluation of some form of treatment. The purely descriptive work has been largely qualitative, trying to describe some 'typical' or 'interesting' person's life 'from the inside' as they themselves see or experience it – the life history interview technique. It is our contention that these methods can also be used to advantage in case evaluation. The quantitative/experimental work has mostly focused on treatment evaluation in the health or social work professions.

A second kind of 'single-case' research involves the description or evaluation of a single setting or the practices within it – a single workplace, for example. Survey or 'open observation' methods such as we described in Chapters 9 and 13 could be used here, but they can also be modified to become more 'collaborative', involving others within the workplace in the planning and evaluation to a much larger extent than is possible in more 'researcher-directed' methods.

Collaborative approaches avoid some of the ethical, practical and emotional problems of research into your own workplace and working practices, but they raise new problems of their own. We discuss them in the final section of this chapter.

We have not set practical exercises in this chapter, but only planning ones, precisely because the way we have chosen to outline these approaches is so bound up with the treatment of cases. We did not think it a good idea to recommend that you try 'interfering in people's lives' just to try out a research technique. Single-case research is a partial way out of one of the great ethical dilemmas of treatment research – the need, purely for the sake of the research design, to withhold a treatment which one suspects is beneficial from some subjects – because when working with single cases there is no control group. Similar problems can occur, nonetheless, particularly in experimental designs. The whole relationship between treatment and research is fraught with ethical problems.

Single-case experimental designs

Schematically, this kind of design can be represented as ABA or perhaps AB1B2B3A – untreated state (A) followed by treatment (B) followed by a period of untreated observation (A), or perhaps untreated state (A) followed by a series of treatments until one appears to work (B1, B2, B3 . . .), followed by a period of observation (A). The problem is in establishing the validity of the conclusion that it *is* the treatment (or something associated with it) which produces the effect. As a logical argument this form of study is obviously weak: it lacks the evidence of the same procedure working on several different people, and it lacks any element of replication – repeating it to see if it works twice (with the inference that if it does not work the second time then the first 'effect' may have been a fluke). The basic form of the superstitious argument lies in an appeal to this kind of experience (I crossed my fingers and the terrible thing failed to happen, so it must not have happened *because* I crossed my fingers – ignoring the many times when one has crossed one's fingers without effect, and the many times that something terrible has happened and might well have happened even if one did cross one's fingers).

A basic element of the single-case experimental design is measurement over time and the comparison of treatment with the state of the subject while untreated. Thus, the simplest kind of project would establish baseline measurements before treatment and then alternate application and withdrawal of treatment – ABABABA . . . In this way the subject acts as 'control' as well as 'treatment' condition – the state when untreated repeatedly acts as a comparison point for the state after treatment. There is variability *within* subjects as well as between them – people differ across time – but by alternating treatments one effectively controls for within-subject variability. It is possible to evaluate different treatments against each other by this means as well, comparing each with the untreated state – $AB_1AB_2AB_3$ . . . (Because the person changes in the course of the treatment series, it would actually be necessary to apply each several times in alternation – AB1AB2AB1AB2 . . .) The argument always rests on the stability of Condition A, the untreated condition, however; the subject may show variation, but this must 'average out'. The basic 'resting state' against which all else is compared must broadly resemble itself from one period of measurement to another (or any trends must be calculable, so that allowance can be made for them).

A second way of overcoming the variability of the individual subject is by frequently repeated measurement. If you were working with a group of subjects you would take a measurement from each of them and average them to get a stable estimate of how the group was proceeding. With the single subject this is not possible, so one has to average over time, which means measurement at more frequent intervals than would be normal in group research. The measurements can then be added together and averaged to give a single reading for a designated time-period which is to some extent free of chance variation because several different readings have gone into it, any of which could by chance have varied in either direction from the average. Repeated measurement over a reasonably long time-period is particularly important at the 'diagnostic' stage, to establish with some reliability the baseline against which the results of treatment(s) are to be judged.

The problem with single-case designs, quite clearly, is establishing validity, reliability and generality without the power to average between subjects to eliminate chance fluctuations and unique events. Repeated and frequent measurement may answer the problem of reliability, the extent to which the measures taken are stable ones, by the direct test of repeating them. Validity may be established by a number of means: validity of measurement by using already validated tests, or by using more than one observer or more than one kind of measure and checking that all show similar trends; validity of design by careful specification of the treatment and careful definition of goals, and by putting great care into establishing that the initial baseline measurements are stable. The question of generalizability is more difficult; it is difficult to generalize from the single subject to a population. Sometimes, where the aim is assessing the results of a particular therapy on the single patient, this may not matter. Often, however, one wishes to be able to say whether a treatment that has succeeded in this case would succeed in others, and if so, then *which* others. The best we can do here is to argue that what works for one subject stands a reasonable chance of working with other 'similar' subjects. Single-case research may be a good way of *building* techniques, but research on groups may be needed to *test* them.

We have stressed the disadvantages of single-case studies, in terms of generalizability. One should realize, however, that there are countervailing disadvantages to studies of groups. The need in an applied setting to work with what is available may lead to very unrepresentative group results; where a 'problem' is not randomly spread through the population, and where a non-random subsection of those coming forward with it actually reach research attention, there is no reason to suppose that an available group is any more representative of the population than a single case. Indeed, because of the

depth in which single cases are studied and the effort which is put into speci-
fying the population of which they may be typical, it can in practice be true
that single-case research is more readily generalizable than more conventional
research carried out on groups.

> The *generality of results* from single-case research is . . . a major issue.
> Concerns often have been voiced about the fact that only one or two
> subjects are studied at a time and the extent to which findings extend to
> other persons is not known. Actually, there is no evidence that findings
> from single-case research are any less generalisable than findings from
> between-group research. In fact, because of the type of interventions
> studied in single-case research, the case is sometimes made that the
> results may be more generalisable than those obtained in between-group
> research.
>
> (Kazdin 1982: 288)

A major check on results, in single-case research as in any other, is replication
– doing the job again. In probability terms, if the probability of a chance
result is low when you do the research once, then the chances multiply
when you do it twice and get the same result. The chance of drawing the King
of Spades from the pack one is 1 in 52. The chances of doing so twice are 1 in
$52 \times 52 = 2704$ – vanishingly small. Where there are doubts of generalizability and of control of sporadic variation, as in single-case designs, replication becomes particularly important. It is for this reason that the ABAB design
is seen as basic to single-case research – it builds in one automatic replication
on the same case. Partial and systematic replication may be used to explore
conceptually distinct aspects of the original successful treatment, by varying
aspects of the original 'package' systematically in subsequent cases.

> Replication can be accomplished in different ways depending on the
> precise aspect of generality in which the investigator is interested. To
> investigate generality across subjects, the investigator can conduct a
> direct replication . . . applying the same procedures across a number of
> different subjects. To evaluate the generality of findings across a variety
> of different conditions . . . the investigator can conduct a systematic
> replication . . . purposely allowing features of the original experiment to
> vary . . . Actually, direct and systematic replications are not qualita-
> tively different. An exact replication is not possible in principle since
> repetition of the experiment involves new subjects tested at different
> points of time and perhaps by different investigators . . . all replications
> necessarily allow some factors to vary.
>
> (Kazdin 1982: 284)

Exercise 34: Planning a single-case experimental design

Develop a plan for research into the treatment of obesity in a single patient. How would you demonstrate validity, reliability and generalizability? What modifications might you need to make to render your design ethically acceptable as research?

There are no right answers to these questions, but our attempts at them may be found at the end of the chapter.

Life history interviewing

At the other extreme of the single-case research design comes the life history interview. Here you pick a single informant and interview repeatedly, exploring the whole of his or her life. You would start off in a comparatively non-directive fashion – perhaps making sure that each segment of the life was covered, and redirecting the informant from what were obviously long and non-productive detours, but otherwise asking little except 'What happened next?' In later interviews you might want to clarify the earlier ones – we are all sometimes inconsistent and even inaccurate in detailing our past lives, and the 'outside eye' of an interviewer can often help to clarify chronology – and to feed back reports of later judgements which are formally inconsistent with reports of earlier ones (as where a particular person is reported as untrustworthy in describing an early stage of life, but as a friend in a later one or *vice versa*). In still later interviews you will be questioning expressed value judgements, to make sure you understand them and their limitations, and posing formal inconsistencies as questions for the informant to rethink. In later interviews again you might be posing the questions which matter to *you* as a researcher/practitioner.

This is the approach which you would undoubtedly use if your field of study were not already well researched, or if you were unhappy with the research and theorization which dominated the field so far. It allows you to carry out research which is holistic and comparatively unfocused. That is, it does not focus in on 'variables', but tries for a complete description of the person's life and how he or she sees the social world. Within this description you hope to find your 'problem' – health attitudes, or growing old and coping, or dealing with heart disease in the family – located and intermeshed with all the other aspects of life and relationship. (If not, a bit of judicious probing will undoubtedly allow you to trace out the relationships.) Even if you propose a survey or experiment at a later date, in an ill-explored field you would undoubtedly start with some form of open, 'qualitative' interviewing and life history interviewing is the form which imposes least structure and preconception on the informant.

It may also be a relevant way of conducting research into practice. What we have talked about so far are treatment-oriented techniques of differing degrees of reductionism and quantitative complexity. Another kind of evaluation of the service you are providing, however, stands back from immediate detail and tries to understand the client's or patient's life as a whole, with your treatment-orientated concerns fading to become just one part, and perhaps not a very large part. Understanding maternity, or old age, or chronic disability or the problems of those caring for sick or disabled dependents might best be approached by this means. It might also give you a better perspective than more focused evaluation on whether the service you provide is effective, or relevant, or even noticed particularly by the informant. More focused evaluation techniques can explore treatment packages and service provision in the terms in which *you* conceive them, but to explore what place they play in the *informant*'s life you need the more open and less pre-structured approach which something like the life-history approach can offer.

The disadvantage – or indeed, perhaps the advantage – of this approach to understanding the informant's life is that it is almost entirely retrospective in its angle of view. You are asking the informant to tell the story of his or her life from now backwards, or from the beginning until now, but in either case it will be told *as it makes sense now*. It will be an account from the point of view of the present, weighted according to the present's concerns and structured to make sense of the present. The informant may on occasion be able to report that 'things seemed different then', but even this is an account of past feeling structured from the point of view of the present. The disadvantage, as with all accounts, is that the past will be 'constructed' to make sense. (This is not because it is the past, but because what we have is an account; an account of the present would be similarly constructed to make sense.) The advantage is that what we learn is not an array of dispassionate 'facts', but that way of structuring the informant's past which demonstrates (or conceals, but makes available for discovery) its impact on present life and attitudes.

Exercise 35: Preparing for life history interviewing

Taking the same theme of obesity, how would you go about conducting a life history interview to cast light on the topic? What sort of person would you want as an informant? How would you approach the task and structure the series of interviews? Under what circumstances might the outcome be relevant for professional practice?

Our attempts at an answer can be found at the end of the chapter.

Collaborative evaluation

Conventionally, research follows one of two models. In academic research, however noble the aims of the researcher, the research can very fairly be described as being in the interests of the researcher: he or she does it to retain an academic job, to obtain promotion, to 'improve the *curriculum vitae*' when it comes to looking for jobs, or for the glory (and, very occasionally, the final profit) of being published. Employed research is generally done in the interests of a customer: the research team is employed to find a solution to a problem. Both kinds of research are fairly charged with using people as objects: the subjects or the research are raw material for academic analysis or commercial or management exploitation. Increasingly, under the influence of both humanistic psychologists and feminists, researchers are turning to a more collaborative way of working, with researchers and other participants all combining to solve some problem which is of importance to the participants, and research reports emerging as a by-product rather than the main aim. The essential issue is one of power: who 'owns' the research, the data and the report?

In this final section of the chapter we look at such 'collaborative' research – research which involves the participants as partners, though not always *equal* partners. Very different kinds of research can be seen as 'collaborative', solving the ethical and power issues in quite different ways. If you are planning collaborative work it is important to be clear what kind of research you are undertaking, and what commitment to and relationship with the researched population it entails. You need to be honest with your informants, and it is equally important to ensure that the 'contract' you have undertaken is capable of being fulfilled and is capable of delivering the kind of research 'product' that you need.

The most collaborative of all research designs comes from the area of psychotherapy, with the concept of co-counselling. Concerned with the power inequality implicit in the therapeutic relationship, some counsellors have adopted a procedure whereby both parties to a therapeutic interview are regarded equally as counsellor and as client – that is, the problems of both are explored, and each attempts to deliver help to the other (see Jackins 1965). On some rare occasions, jointly written research reports have emerged from such projects. More frequently, when such a style of work is deliberately adopted as a *research* tactic, it is to explore some aspect of human feeling or interaction (see, e.g. Heron 1973). Sometimes the research is carried out by a whole interacting group (e.g. Heron 1978), which gives more breadth to the analysis (but makes a truly collaborative write-up more difficult to achieve). Outside the bounds of humanistic psychology some feminist and other 'consciousness-raising' and mutual support groups might fall within this category – those genuinely set up by participants who share a problem and look together for a solution.

Similar approaches have been taken to the assessment and appraisal of professional performance. Teachers, for example, have entered into 'mutual evaluation contracts' wherey they appraised each other's classroom performance and enabled each other to see what they looked like when seen through other eyes, and similar collaborative evaluations have been carried out in the medical profession and in management (see Heron 1977, 1979, 1981). As a feedback method it has great advantages, the chief being that the assessment is not carried out by some outsider standing in a position of potential power over the subject of the appraisal, but by involved colleagues who are themselves to be appraised by the same process.

Not infrequently you will find a piece of research described as co-research whose declared aim is 'facilitation' – helping people to see their situation for what it is. Many feminist papers are of this kind, and some interactional work inspired by a Marxist viewpoint which seeks to teach people about their working situation and the direction in which their interests 'really' lie. Some more humanistic work can also be described in these terms. Note, however, that this kind of 'facilitation' is *not* collaborative in the same way as co-research or collaborative appraisal. It does not exhibit the same equality of power and ownership; on the contrary, its essence is that of one group (researchers) changing or working on another group (subjects/participants). Similar rhetoric does not necessarily guarantee similarly structured research.

A second collaborative model is that of the researcher, as researcher or as social scientist, joining a group's efforts to obtain some shared goal – and, in the process, writing up the struggle towards that goal as a report of research – collaborative action research. Many of the good examples are feminist. For example, Maria Mies and a group of other sociologists, all active in the Women's Movement, helped to obtain a shelter for battered women in Cologne and went on, with the collaboration of those who came to the shelter, to explore women's experiences of being wives under these circumstances (Mies 1983). This differs from the examples above in that the researchers were not directly dealing with a problem which they shared – they had not themselves been in such a relationship (one presumes) – but they made the problem their own and worked along with those who did have direct experience of it to deal with the practical difficulties and the emotional problems experienced by the latter. This kind of research may be seen as collaborative in the sense that it deals with a problem which oppresses the subjects of the research, and they have substantial control over how the campaign and the research associated with it are to be conducted. Power inequality is not totally abolished, however; it is quite clear who are the researchers or sociologists and who are the people with a problem. The question of 'ownership' – whose views are to predominate in any report – is an open one, for negotiation from project to project. Whether the researcher should have the right or power to publish even without the consent of the participants is an important ethical question here.

Slightly more problematic, from the point of view of collaboration, is research in which the researchers have defined the goals and have the task of persuading the 'collaborators' to them as well as carrying out the practical/political task and reporting on it. Again many of the good recent examples are feminist. Some kinds of 'consciousness-raising' groups, for example, would fall in this category – those where an experienced worker sets up a group in order to facilitate change in women's lives. This attachment of researchers' interests to 'subjects' may be more obvious still in some educational projects, where the development of a non-sexist curriculum has been carried through 'collaboratively' whether or not the full population of teachers shares the concept of sexism as a problem.

Slightly further still from the collaborative ideal is the project in which the social intervention is genuinely collaborative – where, for example, the researcher is running a collaborative group as part of his or her normal professional practice – but where the function of the group as research material is concealed from the 'subjects' or at least not their primary concern. Jean Orr's research on the women's groups which she chaired, discussed in an earlier chapter, might be seen as falling in this category: the groups were genuinely run for the benefit of the participants, who were much involved on occasion in how they should be run for this purpose, but Jean's interest in them as a researcher was extraneous to the running of the groups.

A third broad sense of 'collaboration' applies to research where the researcher has been called in (in some sense) to solve a problem by forming and communicating a full understanding of what is going on in the eyes of all parties – a sort of 'communications expert'. Examples would be Elden's work with bank employees, designing and facilitating an on-line computer system to replace existing clerical procedures (Elden 1979, 1981), and Brown and Kaplan (1981) examining working relations and potential for change in a major chemicals plant. In both cases the researcher goes in (with the – sometimes reluctant – backing of management) to explore the situation rather than to prescribe solutions or even to declare the nature of 'the problem'. He or she talks to workers, management, other interested parties, perhaps customers, and tries to build as complete an understanding of the existing situation as possible. Only then does it become possible to define problems (often different problems affecting the different parties), to communicate the nature of each party's problems to the others and finally to work towards solutions. At all stages the researcher obsessively tries not to identify with any particular party. The idea is for the researcher or research team to act like a priest or confidante, someone that all parties can talk to. At the same time the research has an instrumental role, but it is a role primarily dictated by the participants: the researcher is a tool for the communication of information and the resolution of emergent disputes.

Exercise 36: Planning a collaborative exploration

Suppose you had the task of planning a collaborative appraisal (a sort of quality assurance study) of a closed institution – quite a small one, with fifteen or fewer residents, a slow rate or turnover of residents, and about eight or ten staff – how would you go about doing it, and what aims might you set yourself and the project?
    Our answer is at the end of the chapter.

Further reading

Bowles, Gloria and Klein, Renate (eds) (1983). *Theories of Women's Studies*. London: Routledge and Kegan Paul (articles by Klein, Du Bois, Mies, Reinharz, Stanley and Wise, Westcott, Evans).

Hammersley, Martyn and Atkinson, Paul (1989). *Ethnography: Principles in Practice*. London: Routledge.

Hersen, Michael and Barlow, David (1976). *Single-Case Experimental Designs*. Oxford: Pergamon.

Kazdin, Alan (1982). *Single-Case Research Designs*. Oxford: Oxford University Press.

Oja, Saron and Smulyan, Lisa (1988). *Collaborative Action Research*. Basingstoke: Falmer.

Reason, Peter and Rowan, John (eds) (1981). *Human Inquiry: A Sourcebook of New Paradigm Research*. Chichester: Wiley.

Rose, Stephen and Black, Bruce (1985). *Advocacy and Empowerment*. London: Routledge and Kegan Paul.
Smith, Dorothy (1987). *The Everyday World as Problematic*. Boston: Northeastern Universities Press (Section 5, 'Researching the everyday world as problematic').
Williams, Paul and Shoultz, Bonnie (1982). *We Can Speak for Ourselves*. London: Souvenir Press.

Answers to exercises

Exercise 34

What you would do here depends crucially on your theoretical stance. If you are taking a behavioural stance to the problem, you would be focusing on over-eating as a set of habits and looking for weight reduction via control of eating or control of circumstances in which eating takes place. Your 'treatment' might involve making the person aware of how much he or she eats, and how often, by getting him or her to keep a 'food diary' and even perhaps to weigh all food before eating. It might involve a controlled diet, to re-accustom the stomach to being less distended. It might involve identifying the circumstances under which the person 'snacks' and getting him or her to avoid those circumstances, or substituting another activity – walking, listening to music – for the snacking. If you take a more holistic stance you might be looking more to 'underlying factors' which initiate the over-eating – depression or over-strain or some idea of making oneself more or less attractive for some at most half-admitted purpose. Then your treatment might involve counselling – to attack the feelings and self-judgements directly – and an attempt to re-arrange the person's life to make it more rewarding or to substitute other rewards for the rewards of eating.

Whichever, the first stage would have to be a very thorough investigation of the existing situation – how heavy the person is and how the weight fluctuates, what is eaten and when, what the person does during the day, with whom (and with what success) he or she interacts, what demands are placed on him or her, perhaps his or her self-image and beliefs about the self, and his or her feelings and beliefs about food and eating. A goal would be formulated in terms of weight loss and perhaps a change in patterns of social interaction. (The goals would have to be formulated in collaboration with the client – ethically because it is his or her body and his or her life, and practically because the client would be the one actually to 'apply the treatment'.) You would arrange for the client to keep records during the treatment, and times would be assigned for you to visit again to collect information yourself. At regular intervals you would monitor the achievement of the goals and decide whether to discontinue the 'treatment', to continue with it or to change it, and to see whether other problems emerged apart from the one you were 'treating'. At the end, after treatment is discontinued, you would continue to monitor for a while, to ensure that progress was maintained.

You would deliberately alternate periods of treatment and non-treatment – return to previous behaviour – to establish convincingly that it was the treatment that produced the effect. You might well feel that this kind of experiment, with its deliberate reversions to the untreated condition, was not an ethically justified way of proceeding against any problem which really mattered to the client, whether or not consent and collaboration was achieved.

Exercise 35
Here you would be trying for a much broader focus and not working towards treatment at this time – except insofar as the mere act of researching a problem and taking an interest in those who suffer from it has a therapeutic effect in itself, something which has often been found. You would start by getting the informant talking about his or her childhood in general terms, probably, and lead steadily up to the present day and plans for the future. On the way through you would be taking note of anything that emerged about food, meals, poverty, attractiveness or other potentially related topics, but you would probably leave it fairly late in the series of interviews to introduce these deliberately as topics for discussion. At the end you might well find clues as to treatment for this informant or similar informants, in general. For example, using the more structured approach of the Role Repertory Grid, Fay Fransella has examined groups of obese people and also groups of stutterers, eliciting their pictures of themselves and key others in their lives, and also their picture of people who are obese or who stutter (the work is described in Bannister and Fransella 1971). The most interesting thing is that the people with the 'problem' had a quite clear picture of the kind of person who had that problem, but they did not describe themselves in those terms. It was as though, for example, the world were divided into obese people and others, and some of the 'others' (including the informant) happened to eat rather a lot.

Exercise 36
The question describes a project which one of us (Sapsford) is currently carrying out in collaboration with Edna Conlan of Milton Keynes Community Health Council and Milton Keynes Mental Health Advocacy Group. We were first involved in planning the project at the request of the local management of the Unit, with a 'brief' to plan a 'quality auditing system' for the institution. Funding has been obtained from the local health authorities. The scheme which was evolved required a 'baseline study' to set the parameters and establish the system, plus regular 'top-up' research. We rejected quantitative approaches as not appropriate for such a small location, and as incompatible with some of our aims. The major and immediate aim of the project is to identify problems and to monitor the quality of service and how well it fulfils its 'philosophy'. Beyond this, however, lies the hope that the research procedures will themselves help to foster a 'culture of openness' between all the parties involved which will eventually make the research redundant.

At the baseline stage three kinds of 'users' of the institution were to be involved in some depth:

1 The residents – long-stay mental patients mostly being tested out for transfer to some less secure facility. These were to be involved fully in the research: a discussion group will be set up to explain the project to them and start collecting their views of the institution, its philosophy, how it is run and what needs changing (and also what needs preserving). This will be supplemented by individual inter-

views with every resident who is prepared to be interviewed, to get at matters which they do not wish to discuss in public and to give the shy and inhibited a right to have their voices heard.

2 The staff – a general meeting is not practicable, because of staggered shifts and the need for some to be on duty at all times, but all will be interviewed individually.

3 Outside managers, medical authorities, etc. – those who are responsible for sending patients to the institution or who fund or control it: it would not be possible to cover all of these, as the number is potentially very large, but we shall identify about a dozen key figures and interview them.

The baseline study will be written up as a report. Then at 6-monthly intervals we shall hold a further meeting of residents, talk to a sample of staff and write to a sample of outside providers, to see what has changed. More detailed investigation might be undertaken if the results seemed to warrant it – e.g. interviewing all residents. Local problems which emerge would be reported direct to management; more general issues might be raised in a brief annual report. We reserved the right to produce something for a journal, at some stage, describing the project and how it was set up.

☰ Section 4 ☰

In conclusion

15

Writing up

When the research is finished, the data are collected and the analyses done, then the real work starts and you face the question you have been dreading: how to write it up? This chapter looks at what is done in formal research reports, and also at three other modes of presentation – more popular articles, oral presentations and posters. The main issues are the same throughout.

A report or article or lecture has, obviously, to present the facts – what you set out to find, what you found and how you went about finding it. It has to demonstrate the validity of your research and its conclusions – that your research design was appropriate for the purpose and capable of sustaining the results you are claiming, that your measures or data-collection procedures validly cover what you interpret them as covering, that your interpretation of the findings is the best one available. (More to the point, the report makes it possible for other readers to test and question your research and to uncover ways in which it may *not* be valid and ways in which your interpretations may *not* be the only or the best conclusions to be drawn.) Most of all, the report has also to make interesting reading. It has to show why the research was *worth* doing, to tell the story of the fieldwork in an interesting manner and to grip the reader in your final discussion.

The first thing you need is an interesting title – not 'Further research on the on-ward personal interactions of a sample of male patients aged 35–45 in the county of Shropshire', but 'Interaction on the ward: a study of male patients.' However, it should be one that contains enough information to attract relevant readers (in this case 'Interaction' and 'ward/patient' are the key terms). Next in a formal report comes an Abstract, a short (200-word?) summary of what the problem is, what research was done and what the conclusions are. The final version of this is generally written last, although read first, because you can never know quite how the paper will come out until you have written it. In all research writing it is a good stratagem, however, to write a first draft of it as the first thing you write, and to keep it by you as a 'route-map' to what you intend to show, a 'plot' for the story you are going to tell. Next, it is good and pleasant practice to have a brief 'Acknowledgements' section (or to incorporate a paragraph of them into your introduction), thanking those who have helped or advised you. Then you write yourself section headings, and within them you note very briefly what you will want to say in each section and in what order – a more detailed route-map. You get your material – books you want to quote, tables or extracts from interviews, diagrams, etc. – organized for each section. Then you are ready to start.

The rest of this chapter looks at stylistic questions involved in different kinds of report writing. We cannot teach you how to write – this comes with practice. However, in our experience the business of writing is hard (but rewarding) work, so you should not be surprised if you become bored, tired or disorientated. All you can do about this is to keep writing, getting words on paper and hoping that they will 'come out right'. Getting started at all is always difficult, so the best thing once you have planned your route is to plunge straight in and start writing, even if you do not much like what you are writing. The whole paper will undoubtedly need revision before it is presentable – most good papers go through several drafts – and the introductory paragraphs are the most likely of all the sections to need redrafting, so there is little point in trying so hard to get them right first time that you slow yourself down and do not write the rest of the paper. Get the words on paper, even if they are not the right words; revising a rough draft is easier work than writing it in the first place. (There is much to be said for using a word-processor, if you are able: redrafting becomes much easier.) Get someone else to look at and comment on your drafts, and tell them not to be afraid to be rude where necessary; you know what you wanted to get over, but it takes other people to tell you whether you succeeded and where you went wrong.

Formal reports: quantitative research

There is a traditional format which quantitative ('scientific') research reports are supposed to follow – the format which you may have used for writing up physics or chemistry experiments at school. Broadly, the report will fall into clear and labelled sections: Introduction, Methods, Results, and Discussion. The Introduction will set up the area of research and the 'problem' which is to be examined; it may, in fact, run to more than one section, if you have a lot to say and several disparate literatures to review, e.g. Introduction, The Hospital System, Research on Interaction. The Methods section says succinctly, but in enough detail that your methods can be judged by the reader, what you did. It may, again, fall into several sections if what is to be described is complex: e.g. Methods, Sampling, The Questionnaire; or Methods, The Pilot Study, Main Fieldwork. The Results section states what you found, comparatively uncritically – the results put forward as facts, and neither qualified nor commented on beyond what is necessary for an immediate understanding of them. Finally, the Discussion section will:

1 restate the findings and explain what they mean in the context of the themes you announced in your Introduction;

2 look at potential weaknesses of the methods and either discount them
   or argue the extent to which the results can be trusted despite these
   weaknesses;
3 outline the implications for the academic area and/or for policy;
4 possibly make recommendations;
5 possibly outline further research that needs to be done.

The length of the whole depends on the outlet through which you intend to
publish it. Psychology journals typically publish articles of 3000–5000 words
(12–20 pages of typescript, double spaced). Sociology journals expect something rather longer – typically 7000–10 000 words. Either may have a 'Brief
Reports' section in which articles of not more than about 2000 words may be
published. You need to look at your target publication and see what length of
article they expect. An 'internal' report, for a funding authority or your own
management, for example, might be of any length, but typically it would be
rather fuller and more detailed than a journal article. On the other hand, it
would almost certainly start with a one- or two-page section outlining the
main conclusions and recommendations, for those who did not have the time
or expertise to deal with the details.

In the Results section (and elsewhere, if appropriate) you will be presenting
numerical information, often in the form of tables or graphs. It is important
that every factual statement you make is backed up with figures, and unless the
figures are very simple indeed – e.g. a comparison of two percentages or two
means – then will be appropriate to present them in tabular form. The tables
which are presented in the text should form part of the argument and should
be extremely simple and readable – as simple as it as possible to be and still
make the desired point. There may be a case for presenting more complex
figures from which other researchers can check your conclusions or carry out
further analysis, but such 'storehouse' tables should usually be in an Appendix, not in the main text. At the same time you should remember that no set of
figures speaks for itself, and you should always interpret the results in words
as well as giving the figures. Each stage of the argument in the Results section
has the same structure:

1 what is to be shown;
2 how it is to be shown;
3 table or description of results;
4 what it means.

The other requirement, in this kind of research, is that no conclusion should
go *untested*. Wherever you present a result – a difference, or a correlation, or
some other relationship – you should also present an associated test of significance (unless the result is so small or so large that it clearly does not need
testing). You need to show that what you are stating as 'fact' is not a chance
product of sampling variation, so tests of statistical significance are absolutely
required. (Again you should interpret them in words; you cannot safely
assume that all your readers will understand them – particularly if your

Report is for Management or for a funding body.) Even when comparing figures not at first sight based on samples – e.g. the actual numbers of cases processed in two different years – it may still be appropriate to test for significance, treating the 2 years as random samples from all the years you could possibly have examined and looking for indications of more than chance variation between them.

An important point to remember is that any explicit or implicit promises of confidentiality or anonymity that you have made should be honoured. It is important that your informants should not be identifiable from your report unless they have explicitly stated that their names may be given. To preserve confidentiality may mean going beyond suppressing names, to omitting or changing (fictionalizing) identifiable circumstances.

Formal reports: qualitative research

Qualitative research reports – reports of open interviewing project and/or open or participant observation – do not generally follow this set structure. Researchers of this kind do not generally think of themselves as scientists, and they have no desire to emulate the report of the scientific experiment. However, just the same topics and sections have to be covered in the report. You still have:

1 to introduce your field of research and explain why it is interesting;
2 to explain what you did, and how;
3 to give the results;
4 to interpret them and qualify them.

There is more lee-way to 'tell the story', but you still have to demonstrate that what you did was a valid way of researching the problem or area you elected to tackle, and that your interpretation of what was said to you and what you saw is a valid one. Thus, without having the same formal sub-headings, you may well find yourself falling into the same general structure.

The presentation of data will necessarily be more impressionistic in this kind of report. Where statements are being made about *numbers* of people who do or say something, tables may still be appropriate, and certainly numbers are better than vague impressions: '60 per cent of the sample' or '90 per cent' carries more conviction and is more interpretable than 'many' or 'a majority'. Often, however, you will be making points about interviews that could be fully substantiated only by reproducing the entire transcript, which is not practical for reasons of length and because the point would still not emerge until the reader had put as much time into analysis as you have done. One therefore makes points and illustrates them with pertinent quotations from the transcript. One or two quotations do not constitute compelling evidence, but they give a feel for what the informant actually said and allow the reader to try interpreting it in some different way.

A key aspect of validating qualitative research is *reflexivity* – showing at each stage of the report that you have a reasonable grasp of what went on, how

you were seen and construed by the informant(s) and the extent to v
own preconceptions, theoretical frame or professional status may !
acted with the data and your interpretation of it. Hitting the righ
reflexivity is difficult. If your report reads too much like a diary of your
feelings and experiences and is too dominated by 'I', 'me' and 'my', it will
annoy or embarrass the reader. On the other hand, this kind of research is
mediated through the person of the researcher, and we need to find out about
that person in order to understand and trust the results. This is very much a
case for showing your first draft to someone else – preferably someone experienced in this kind of research – to see if you have hit the right level.

In reports of this kind of research we need to remember that it is the detail
that carries conviction, but that the detail is also what can betray the identity
of the informants. Particular care must be exercised that people are not
'exposed' in this way, so fictional names are normally given to informants and
it is often necessary to suppress or even fictionalize some of the details, or to
'add two cases together', in order not to publish the intimate details of an identifiable individual's life.

Other modes of presentation

Quite often what you are called on to write is not a formal research report, but
a 'popular account', by which we mean anything from an account for the
general public to an article in a professional journal aimed more at practice
than research (e.g. *Nursing Times*, *Social Work Today*). The same considera-
tions come into play – you must still give enough detail of how the research
was carried out that its validity can be judged by the informed reader. However, the 'slant' will necessarily be different, more towards why the area is
interesting and how your results contribute to it, and less towards the detail of
the research procedures. You can allow yourself a greater degree of specula-
tion and 'following up ideas' in a popular account than would be normal in a
formal report. However, you should never state as fact (or imply to be true)
what you have not established, and you should be very careful about over-
generalizing your results and claiming for the research an importance which it
does not bear.

A more difficult task which you may well be called on to perform if you have
carried out research is to make an oral presentation – a lecture, or a short
presentation, to a public audience or your peers or to management or those
who have commissioned or funded the research. The same principles apply,
but your presentation has to be less dense, with only the important highlights
brought out. You would be surprised how little can be delivered in a given
amount of time when you present your results orally. You will be lucky to get
one 'point' across in 5 minutes in a compressed and 'slick' session such as a
market-research presentation, and in the more relaxed and didactic setting of
a lecture one point in ten minutes would be more realistic. This means that you
can only say five or six things in an hour's lecture, and you have to be very
careful and self-disciplined in selecting the six points that you want to make.

Time is saved, and the pace of the presentation is more enjoyable for the audience, if you use pre-prepared visual aids such as slides for an overhead projector. These can be used to present tables and diagrams, and also to summarize lists to points in a memorable form. Photocopied 'hand-outs' can also be used, to deliver material which it is essential for the audience to receive, but which does not fit easily within the ambit of the lecture (i.e. detailed tables or details of controversial aspects of the research process).

Finally, at conferences and other situations where research results are exchanged, there is a growing fashion for 'poster' presentation – researchers delivering their results in visual form, often literally on one poster (but being present to discuss them with anyone whom the poster attracts). The skill here, obviously, is the skill of Abstract-writing – working out the absolute minimum that needs to be displayed, and presenting it in a graphic and arresting form (with at least some important part of it readable from a distance). You can make even fewer points than in a lecture, and they have to be made in a very few words or, preferably, pictorially. Sometimes cartoons can be used to advantage. For an example of a research project whose report was presented in this way, see the article 'Doing dialogical research' by Rosemary Randall and John Southgate, in Reason and Rowan (1981).

Exercise 37: Writing up

If you would like to, why not take one of the small pieces of research you carried out in connection with Chapter 1 – perhaps the structured and unstructured observation – and try writing it up? (Look at some examples of reports first – see below.) Aim for something quite short – 2000 words at most. Get someone familiar with research to look over it and comment on it for you. Then think how you could boil it down to (a) a 20-minute oral presentation, and (b) a poster display.

Further reading

For examples of quantitative reports, see the articles by Abbott and Payne, Choon and Skevington, Gordon, and Dingwall and Fox, in Abbott and Sapsford (eds) (1992) *Research into Practice: A Reader for Nurses and the Caring Professions*. The Gordon article is probably the best to use as a model, in terms of structure.

For examples of qualitative reports, see the articles by Kirkham and by Abbott and Sapsford, in the same book.

16

In conclusion

Section 3 of this book was mostly about techniques and approaches. In this final chapter we should like to look further at what lies *behind* the research which you carry out or read about. Research is seldom or never carried out just 'to collect the facts' in some supposedly neutral way. Behind the research project lies the hypothesis to be tested, the theory to be extended or clarified, the problem to be solved, the policy to be evaluated, the practice to be improved or monitored. Even the Census is not a totally neutral piece of data-collection; the questions which are chosen are there because answers are *needed* – for planning schools, hospitals, local services, etc. We may divide research projects and programmes, crudely, into those which are aimed at the development and elucidation of theory ('academic research') and those which are aimed at solving a practical problem, or developing or monitoring a social policy, or assessing and improving how professionals or others do their jobs ('applied research'). This chapter is structured as if the divide between these two kinds of research were an absolute one. As we shall see, however, theory and practice interpenetrate – theory has consequences, and practice is based explicitly or implicitly on theory.

Research into practice

'Applied research' is not one kind of thing, but many. It ranges from the immediate and local evaluation of a particular treatment or change of working practice which you yourself are thinking of adopting, through evaluating your practice as a whole, evaluating the practice of a group of people, assessing the work of a unit or an institution, or evaluating the success of a policy which rules over a wide range of institutions, to large-scale fact-finding exercises on which policy may be based. Some common themes run through all of these kinds of work, however. In all of them it is necessary to specify the 'problem' with great care, to define with precision the goal of the policy or practice or innovation, and to specify what shall count as a favourable or unfavourable outcome. In thinking about outcomes it is necessary to use a great deal of imagination, to get beyond the formal 'declaration of purpose' and think how the policy-makers or practitioners will react to various kinds of outcome which they have not yet envisaged (and the same applies when you are setting out to evaluate your own practice). It is necessary also to think carefully about the way that the research is framed and the way in which you intend to carry it out, to see who might be hurt or unsettled by it and whose interests might be harmed.

Assessing a new way of nursing certain patients, for instance, the declared goal will undoubtedly be to improve the health or speed the recovery of the patients; we are all in favour of honour and virtue, and the virtuous nurse works towards the good of the patients. Thinking of what outcomes would be *acceptable*, however, we would probably feel that the technique was worth introducing if it made the patients more comfortable, or even if they just preferred it to the previous way of working, even if it had no measurable effect on health. We might even think it worth introducing if all it did was to make the nurse's job easier or more pleasant, provided the patients were no worse off than before. So an acceptable outcome may be something substantially less than would be implied by the rhetoric of treatment. We have also to consider the *constraints* on acceptability. If we carried out research on a nursing treat- ment and found it had a measurable effect on speed of recovery, we might declare the treatment a success. Would it be adopted, however, if it cost a great deal more than the previous treatment? Or if it meant substantially increasing the establishment of nursing staff? Or if it meant a great deal more work for the nurses who implemented it? *How much* extra cost, in money or staff or time, would be acceptable? In other words, is the goal better formulated as 'to speed recovery, or to make patients more comfortable, *at little or no extra cost*'? Indeed, might it be true (as often appears the case at the time of writing) that the real goal is to reduce costs, with the constraint being that patients must not be much worse off and nurses not much more hard pressed in their jobs? The true goals of policy-makers (or your own, looking at your own practice) may not be as honourable and virtuous as the usual rhetoric may suggest.

The difference between rhetoric and reality is well worth bearing in mind when reading other people's research. Sometimes you will find that apparent lapses of logic – rejecting conclusions on less than adequate grounds, or jumping to conclusions as 'obvious' which seem less than obvious to you – may betray a 'hidden agenda' influenced by what is implicitly counted as an adequate outcome or implicitly acknowledged as a constraint on the accept- ability of an outcome, without the writer having explicitly stated what is affecting his or her judgement. Indeed, you may come across the occasional report which quite blatantly reinterprets the evidence, not to assess whether current practice fits the declared aims, but to show how the declared aims can be reinterpreted to fit current practice. The *status quo* often attracts very powerful defensive manoeuvres.

An important part of 'research imagination' is seeing beyond what one tends to take for granted, looking for different ways of doing what has always been done in a particular way, even questioning whether the reasons why it is done are still beyond questioning. One is reminded of one of the early 'time and motion' studies, carried out on gun-teams in the French army before the Second World War. The researchers worked out what each person in the team was supposed to be doing while the gun was being readied, and it turned out that the entire job of one team member was to hold the officer's horse. French artillery officers had not been mounted for several years by this time.

The taken for granted can readily extend to the perspective from which the research is undertaken. We have talked about ethics throughout this book mainly in terms of avoiding harm to 'subjects', and the question of the extent to which it is legitimate to deceive people and/or use them as 'objects'. Ethical questions also stretch, however, to the perspective from which the research is undertaken. As a practitioner, or as a researcher commissioned by 'management', one naturally feels that the purposes of the system under investigation and the way in which it is run are in the interests of patients/clients/recipients. It is possible, however, that the way these interests are perceived are management-defined, and that the people themselves might define their interests in quite different ways. A case in point is the way in which contraceptive advice is given to black women: we generally accept as liberal and beneficial that advice on contraceptives be made freely available to working-class women. Sometimes black women feel, however, that the advice is aimed mainly at controlling their fertility because of white middle-class fears, and sometimes the evidence suggests that they are right (see Bryan *et al.* 1985, for a discussion). The question of 'neutrality' in research is not an easy one. Clearly, the researcher should not 'take sides' to the extent that the research becomes polemic and results contrary to the researcher's position cannot emerge. We might also argue, however, that one role of social research is to make space for the voices to be heard of those who do not usually get a hearing. If researchers do not in some sense 'speak for the underdog' then it is not clear who will do so (nor why 'the underdog' should tolerate being researched).

Research and theory

By 'theory' in this section we shall mean not the particular theory (derived perhaps from sociology or social psychology) which a programme of research might be designed to test, but underlying perspectives or models (of the social order and the nature of people and institutions within it) which are expressed in the way the research is conceptualized. Again, we are looking critically at what is taken for granted, assumed or posited as a natural or sensible way of conceptualizing the world within which the research problem is set.

Models of the social world differ widely. You may conceptualize the social order in a 'functionalist' way, influenced knowingly or unknowingly by theorists such as Merton and Parsons, and conceive of society as a relatively coherent whole sharing a large measure of agreement as to what is normal and how things should be, but with small pockets of deviants at the outskirts who do not or cannot share that consensus. In that case your conception of the research problem is likely to be influenced by the notion that every social structure has a function – by definition, because in this view a structure which was not functional would not survive – and be interested in working out what that function was. (The concept of 'the sick role' is a typical functionalist notion.) You may hold an essentially Marxist or 'conflict theory' model of society, seeing the social order as riven with economic inequalities, and social structures as set up to maintain and promote the position of the dominant class (those who own or control the means of production). Concepts of ideology are natural in this perspective, and the sort of research that follows from it demonstrates differential health chances by class, or differential use of and benefit from health resources; some of the best research on third world countries, and the role of multi-national drug companies in exploiting markets within them has also been influenced by this perspective. You may find yourself with an essentially individualistic model of the social order, which denies the existence of 'society' or 'social structures' and attempts to explain everything in terms of the interactions of individuals. In addition, or instead, you may be influenced by one of a variety of feminist perspectives, all of which stress the concept of patriarchy or patriarchal relations – the structural and/or personal domination of women by men. Each of these ways of looking at social relations has its impact on how you conceptualize research into the health and personal social services, which lie at an important point of intersection between different theories. How they are conceptualized affects not only how they are expected to function, but also what is likely to be seen as problematic about them.

At the same time a piece of research will entail a model of what people are like. At one extreme the form of conceptualization may embody a variety of determinism, treating people as the product of their inherent nature (biological determinism) or their immediate surroundings (environmental determinism, or behaviourism) or the history and structure of the social order (sociological determinism). At the other extreme, research may conceptualize people as free and autonomous agents (voluntarism) – the thinking, feeling, experiencing beings of some humanistic social psychology, or the imperfect, selfish and competing animals of some New Right conceptualizations. In between come notions of unconscious motivation, ideological influence, and a wide range of theories (interacting with the models of society outlined above) which look for interaction or articulation between the ways in which we may be conceived of as 'free' to decide and the ways in which we may be shown to be 'bound' and determined by factors extrinsic to our consciousness.

Models of the person are strongly reflected in the general styles into which research studies fall. Much quantitative, positivistic research assumes the person as in some way determined, a product of biology or upbringing or environment or social structure. It looks for the causes of events and behaviours, applying consistent stimuli in the assurance of eliciting consistent responses. Some qualitative work embodies a deterministic perspective, but it sees people as the product of their *social* environment – the people around them, the local consensus on norms and values, and/or wider social structures or ideologies. Some qualitative work, still deterministic, is framed in terms of 'inner forces' of which the conscious person may be unaware. Yet other kinds are framed in terms of actually or potentially autonomous people capable of understanding their lives and taking control of them. In all these varieties there is less interest in the supposed causes of behaviours, and more interest in the understanding and analysis of what aspects of the social or individual world *mean* for those who experience them.

A particular conflict of models – not a controversy, but something built into the basic way of looking at things – crops up when we try to do research which is in any sense collaborative and includes the 'subjects' or 'informants' as equal participants. Basic to the notion of collaborative research is a model of all people – not just the researcher – as knowledgeable about their own prob-lems or at least prepared to explore what they may be in the same way as the researcher is prepared to explore them. In other words, the collaborative model assigns no particular expertise or knowledge to the researcher, over and above what he or she may happen to have read. The essence of the collabora-tive approach is that the researcher does not 'own' the research – that he or she is not, in fact, 'the researcher', but merely someone with particular skills or knowledge of literature who is prepared to share these skills. There is a further corollary, that this is how research *should* be, that any other way of approach-ing research is exploitative. This model is central to collaborative research of any kind; to the extent that it does not describe what was going on, the research was not collaborative. On the other hand, there is an in-built tension, in that many who would espouse this style would also believe that we are not free to understand our situation except through education and 'consciousness-raising': that people are deceived by the ideology inherent in their situation and need help to see beyond it. This tension between education and equal participation is entirely typical of collaborative research and is the source of many of its practical and ethical dilemmas.

The 'teaching' point we are trying to make from all this, however, is that *there is no possibility of escaping the effect of underlying models of society and of the person*. To the extent that we try to do 'value-free' research which has no political overtones and just looks to describe 'the facts', we impose common-sense models of society and the person on our research. The disadvantage of the common sense approach – what 'stands to reason' or is seen as 'natural' – is that it is unanalysed. It *may* fairly represent what is going on. It may equally be prone to every ideological and habitual short-cut for avoiding disquieting analysis that the social setting may happen to offer at the time of the research. It is difficult enough to separate oneself from the presuppositions of 'manage-ment'. To separate oneself from one's own presuppositions is more difficult still, and yet it is an essential part of the 'research imagination'.

Most difficult of all to separate oneself from is the set of assumptions built into our everyday thought. We are not speaking here of ideologies – coherent attempts to present someone else's interests as one's own – but what Foucault and others have called 'discourses'. A 'discourse' is a way of speaking about things, a way of 'dividing up the ground'; however, the terms of the discourse are seldom value-neutral. What a discourse does is to 'capture the agenda', to declare what shall be taken for granted as important. When you feel that there is something wrong with a line of argument, but you find it difficult to put it into words, because the terms of the argument do not seem to lend themselves to your way of seeing things and you find yourself arguing 'against the self-evident', this is a sure sign that a conflict of discourses is taking place.

We might illustrate what we mean by discourse from the rhetoric surrounding any General Election – the fight over whether taxation or economic success or defence capability or sensibility to the plight of the poor is to be seen as the mark of 'good government'. Another particularly good example may be built around the concept of family, and the life and life-rights of women. Women may be defined in any one of a set of discourse-laden terms.

1 *Women as wives* clearly have a 'duty to their husbands' – and the duty has sexual implications. The role of a 'wife' is to be an adjunct to her husband, which has strong implications for the place of women in the labour market.
2 *Women as mothers* clearly have a 'duty to their children' – and this duty may interfere with their sexual duty as wives. It is axiomatic that the welfare of children comes before all else, so that this way of viewing women also has strong implications for the place of women in the labour market.
3 *Women as adults* can be seen as having just the same rights and responsibilities as men as adults, including the right to work. However,
4 *Women as workers* have available to them a labour market which takes for granted that they will be constrained by their role as mothers and wives (nurturant, caring, willing and *inherently able* to take on a supportive role). It also takes for granted, largely, that they will be supported by some man and not in need of a 'family wage'. Thus, the mostly female segment of the labour market is very different from the mostly male segment.

In other words, these are incompatible ways of framing the debates: what seems reasonable to say when talking about women as adults (equal citizens) somehow seems to make no sense when talking about women as mothers (people devoted to the care of children).

There is an inherent problem here in what is required of the good researcher. On the one hand, we are required to identify what is taken for granted in the way that problems are formulated for us (in the case of commissioned research) or by us (in the case of research which we ourselves initiate), and in the answers which our informants give us. It is our job to see behind the easy formulation of the problem to the questions that *might* have been asked, and behind the easy answer to questions to the answers that *might* have been given. At the same time, we are people of our own culture, class, gender, race, profession, etc., and it is unclear just *how* we are expected to see behind our preconceptions.

There is no simple or conclusive answer to this question, just as there is no simple or final way of doing the 'seeing behind'. There are two points which might give us hope, however.

1 That there is no single 'discourse' – no single set of concepts which 'describe reality' – but a multiplicity of ways of framing the world. In the example above, for instance, we can conceptualize women as wives, as mothers and as adults, all different ways of structuring the social world with regard to gender, and the fact that there are these different ways allows us to some extent to stand back from all of them.

2 To the extent that we are 'determined' or 'caused' by the prevailing frames, this causal force may be 'quasi-causal' (Wellmer 1969; Sapsford and Thomas 1985) – determining only to the extent that we are not aware of it. The whole force of the idea of 'consciousness-raising' is that what seems natural and is normally taken for granted may be set aside (to some small extent at least) once we realize that there are other ways of formulating the problem. This kind of raising of consciousness is characteristic of the very best outcomes of the research process.

In conclusion

In conclusion, research is not some mysterious 'technical subject' to be mastered by years of study, but something which we all can do and all do in fact *do*. Research is asking questions, looking to see what is going on, trying out what happens if we make this or that change. There *are* techniques, and it helps to know them, but they can all be mastered when they are needed – or you can obtain help from others who *do* know them (e.g. statisticians, computer experts) provided you know *about* them. The more research you do and read about, the more techniques you will know about and have in your 'toolbox' for planning the next project. The key to good research, however, does not lie in the techniques. Good research is the product of clear analysis of problems, clear specification of goals, careful design of fieldwork and thoughtful analysis and exposition afterwards. What lies between is just good, honest work.

At the same time, good research is something very difficult to achieve. It takes a very clear and logical mind, coupled with a great deal of imagination. You have to be able to see round your own taken for granted presuppositions, and those of other people, to find the most fruitful way to formulate the problem and the goals of the research. You have to think clearly about what could possibly be concluded from the data you intend to collect, what objections might be raised to these conclusions, and whether your procedures could be modified to increase the interpretability of the results and to overcome the likely objections. You need great insight into how people will react and a lively apprehension of what could harm them or cause them discomfort. You need the ability to put your own interpretation of the world aside and take on that of the informants, for the purpose of the research, while staying sufficiently marginal to it that it does not dominate your thinking entirely. Finally, you need to be able to put aside your preferred conclusions if the data do not bear them out. All of this is very difficult, and no one ever manages to achieve all of it. It is the goal, however, and most of us occasionally achieve some small part of it.

A final point is that research, as an attitude of mind, is not confined to methods classes and formal research projects. The attitude of mind which is needed for research is also needed for our day-to-day practice. The same principles which inform the major research project also inform our constant small-scale attempts to evaluate and improve our own practice.

Further reading

Abbott, Pamela and Wallace, Claire (1990). *An Introduction to Sociology: Feminist Perspectives*. London: Routledge.
Bannister, Don and Fransella, Fay (1980). *Inquiring Man*. Harmondsworth: Penguin.
Barrett, Michele (1988). *Women's Oppression Today*, 2nd ed. London, Verso.
Billig, Michael *et al.* (1988). *Ideological Dilemmas: A Social Psychology of Everyday Thinking*. London: Sage.
Bryan, Beverley *et al.* (1985). *The Heart of the Race*. London: Virago.
Commission for Racial Equality (1978). *Five Views of Multi-racial Britain*. London: CRE/BBC.
Pryce, Ken (1979). *Endless Pressure*. Harmondsworth: Penguin.
Shotter, John (1975). *Images of Man in Psychological Research*. London: Methuen.
Smith, Dorothy (1987). *The Everyday World as Problematic*. Boston: Northeastern Universities Press.

References

Abbott, Pamela (1982). 'Towards a Social Theory of Mental Handicap'. PhD thesis, Thames Polytechnic.

Abbott, Pamela (ed.) (1988). *Material Deprivation and Health Status in the Plymouth Health District*. Plymouth: Polytechnic South West, Department of Applied Social Science.

Abbott, Pamela and Payne, Geoff (1992). 'Hospital visiting on two wards', in R. Sapsford and P. Abbott (eds) op. cit.

Abbott, Pamela and Sapsford, Roger (1986). 'Diverse reports: caring for mentally handicapped children in the community' *Nursing Times*, 5 March, 47–9.

Abbott, Pamela and Sapsford, Roger (1987a). *Women and Social Class*. London: Tavistock.

Abbott, Pamela and Sapsford, Roger (1987b). *Community Care for Mentally Handicapped Children*. Milton Keynes: Open University Press. (Part is reprinted in Pamela Abbott and Roger Sapsford, op. cit 1992.)

Abbott, Pamela and Sapsford, Roger (1991). 'Health visiting: policing the family?', in P. Abbott and C. Wallace (eds) A *Sociology of the Caring Professions*. Basingstoke: Falmer.

Abbott, Pamela and Sapsford, Roger (eds) (1992). *Research into Practice: A Reader for Nurses and the Caring Professions*. Buckingham: Open University Press.

Abbott, Pamela and Wallace, Claire (1990). *An Introduction to Sociology: Feminist Perspectives*. London: Routledge.

Abbott, Pamela, Bernie, Joyce, Payne, Geoff and Sapsford, Roger (1992). 'Health and material deprivation in Plymouth', in Pamela Abbott and Roger Sapsford (eds) op. cit.

Adelman, Clem and Alexander, Robin (1982). *The Self-evaluating Institution: Practice and Principles in the Management of Educational Change*. London: Methuen.

Anastasi, Anne (1982). *Psychological Testing*. London: Macmillan.

Backett, Kathryn (1982). *Mothers and Fathers*. London: Macmillan.

Bannister, Don and Fransella, Fay (1980). *Inquiring Man: The Theory of Personal Constructs*. Harmondsworth: Penguin.

Barrett, Michele (1988). *Women's Oppression Today: The Marxist/Feminist Encounter*, 2nd edn. London: Verso.

Bayley, Michael (1973). *Mental Handicap and Community Care*. London: Routledge and Kegan Paul.

Billig, Michael *et al.* (1988). *Ideological Dilemmas: A Social Psychology of Everyday Thinking*. London: Sage.

Boulton, Mary (1983). *On Being a Mother*. London: Tavistock.

Bowles, Gloria and Klein, Renate (eds) (1983). *Theories of Women's Studies*. London: Routledge and Kegan Paul.

Breakwell, Glynnis, Foot, Hugh and Gilmour, Robin (eds) (1982). *Social Psychology: A Practical Manual* London: Macmillan/BPS.

Brown, Dave and Kaplan, Robert (1981). 'Participative research in a factory', in P. Reason and J. Rowan (eds) op. cit.

Brown, George and Harris, Tirril (1978). *Social Origins of Depression: A Study of Psychiatric Disorder in Women*. London: Routledge and Kegan Paul.

Brown, Roswyn (1989). *Individualised Care: The Role of the Ward Sister*. Harrow: Scutari.

Bryan, Beverley, Dadzie, Stella and Scafe, Fay (1985). *The Heart of the Race: Black Women's Lives in Britain* London: Virago.

Burgess, Robert (1984). *In the Field: An Introduction to Field Research*. London: Allen and Unwin.

Burns, R.B. (1977). 'Male and female perceptions of their own and other sex' *British Journal of Social and Clinical Psychology*, 16: 213–20.

Busfield, Joan (1991). *Women and Mental Health*. London: Macmillan.

Campbell, D.T. (1969). 'Reforms as experiments' *American Psychologist*, 24: 409–29.

Campbell, D.T. and Ross, H.L. (1968). 'The Connecticut crackdown: time-series data in quasi-experimental analysis' *Law and Society Review*, 3 : 33–53.

Cartwright, A. (1979). *The Dignity of Labour?* London: Tavistock.

Caudill, W., Redlich, F.C., Gilmore, H. and Brody, E.B. (1952). 'Social structure and interaction processes on a psychiatric ward' *American Journal of Orthopsychiatry*, 22: 314–34.

Cavendish, Ruth (1982). *Women on the Line*. London: Routledge and Kegan Paul.

Central Statistical Office (periodically). *Guide to Official Statistics*. London: HMSO.

Choon, George and Skevington, Suzanne (1984). 'How do women and men in nursing perceive each other?', in S. Skevington (ed.) *Understanding Nurses: The Social Psychology of Nursing*. Chichester: Wiley.

Clark, June (1981). *What do Health Visitors do?* London: Royal College of Nursing.

Clegg, Frances (1982). *Simple Statistics*. Cambridge: Cambridge University Press.

Commission for Racial Equality (1978). *Five Views of Multi-racial Britain*. London: CRE/BBC.

Cope, David (1981). *Organisational Development and Action Research in Hospitals*. Aldershot: Gower.

Cornwell, Jocelyn (1984). *Hard-Earned Lives: Accounts of Health and Illness from East London*. London: Tavistock.

Davis, Fred (1963). *Passage through Crisis: Polio Victims and their Families*. Indianapolis: Bobbs-Merril.

Dingwall, Robert (1977). *The Social Organisation of Health Visitor Training*. London: Croom Helm.

Dingwall, Robert and Fox, Susan (1986). 'Health visitors' and social workers' perceptions of child care problems', in A. While (ed.) *Research in Preventive Community Nursing Care: Fifteen Studies in Health Visiting*. Chichester: Wiley. (A slightly shortened version is reprinted in Abbott and Sapsford, op. cit., 1992)

Dixon, Penelope (1967). 'Reduced Emotional Responsiveness in Schizophrenia'. PhD thesis, University of London.

Dominelli, Lena and McLeod, Eileen (1989). *Feminist Social Work*. London: Macmillan.

Drennan, Vari (1986). 'Talking to health visitors – perceptions of their work', in A. While (ed.) *Research in Preventive Community Nursing Care*. Chichester: Wiley.

Elden, Max (1979). 'Bank employees begin to participate in studying and changing their organisation', in International Organisation for the Quality of Working Life *Working on the Quality of Working Life*. The Hague: Martinus Nijhoff.

Elden, Max (1981). 'Sharing the research work: participative research and its role demands', in P. Reason and J. Rowan (eds) op. cit.

Fearn, R. (1987). 'Rural health care: a British success or a tale of unmet need?' *Social Science and Medicine*, 24: 263–74.

Fransella, Fay and Frost, K. (1977). *On being a Woman*. London: Tavistock.

Fulani, Lenora (ed.) (1988). *The Politics of Race and Gender in Therapy*. New York: Haworth Press.

Giovannoni, J.M. and Becerra, R.M. (1979). *Defining Child Abuse*. London: Collier-Macmillan.

Glaser, Barry and Strauss, Anselm (1967). *The Discovery of Grounded Theory*. Chicago: Aldine.

Glendinning, Carolyn (1983). *Unshared Care: Parents and their Disabled Children*. London: Routledge and Kegan Paul.

Goffman, Erving (1961). *Asylums: Essays on the Social Situation of Mental Patients and Other Inmates*. New York: Anchor Books (also Harmondsworth: Penguin).

Goffman, Erving (1963). *Stigma: The Management of Spoilt Identities*. New York: Anchor Books (also Harmondsworth: Penguin).

Gordon, Verona (1982). 'Themes and cohesiveness observed in depressed women's support group' *Issues in Mental Health Nursing*, 4: 115–25.

Gordon, Verona (1986). 'Treatment of depressed women by nurses in Britain and the USA', in J. Brooking (ed.) *Psychiatric Nursing Research*. Chichester: Wiley. (An abridged version is reprinted in Abbott and Sapsford, op. cit., 1992.)

Gordon, Verona and Ledray, L. (1984). 'The alleviation of subclinical depression in women of middle years' (unpublished).

Hammersley, Martyn and Atkinson, Paul (1989). *Ethnography: Principles in Practice*. London: Routledge.

Haskey, John (1989). 'Families and households of the ethnic minority and white populations of Great Britain' *Population Trends*, 57: 8–19.

Heron, John (1973). *Re-evaluation Counselling: A Theoretical Review*. Guildford: University of Surrey Human Potential Research Project.

Heron, John (1977). *Behaviour Analysis in Education and Training*. Guildford: University of Surrey Human Potential Research Project.

Heron, John (1978). *An ASC Peer Research Group*. Guildford: University of Surrey Human Potential Research Project.

Heron, John (1979). *Peer Review Audit*. Guildford: University of Surrey Human Potential Research Project.

Heron, John (1981). 'Self and peer assessment for managers', in T. Boydell and M. Pedler (eds.) *Handbook of Management Self Development*. London: Gower.

Hersen, Michael and Barlow, David (1976). *Single-Case Experimental Designs: Strategies for Studying Behavioural Change*. Oxford: Pergamon.

Hindess, Barry (1973). *The Use of Official Statistics in Sociology*. London: Macmillan.

Hollander, Edwin (1981). *Principles and Methods of Social Psychology*. Oxford: Oxford University Press.

Hollway, Wendy (1989). *Subjectivity and Method in Psychology: Gender, Meaning and Science*. London: Sage.

Home Office (annual). *Statistics of Death Reported to Coroners*. London: HMSO.

Hyener, R.H. (1985). 'Some guidelines for the phenomenological analysis of interview data' *Human Problems*, 8: 279–303.

Irvine, John, Miles, Ian and Evans, Jeff (eds) (1979). *Demystifying Social Statistics*. London: Pluto Press.

Jackins, H. (1965). *The Human Side of Human Beings: The Theory of Re-evaluation Counselling*. Seattle: Rational Island Publishers.

James, Nicky (1984). 'A postscript to nursing', in C. Bell and H. Roberts (eds) *Sociological Research: Politics, Problems, Practice*. London: Routledge and Kegan Paul. (A slightly shortened version is reprinted in Abbott and Sapsford, op. cit., 1992.)

Jensen, Arthur (1981). *Straight Talk about Mental Tests*. London: Macmillan.

Johnson I.S. *et al.* (1987). *Health Care and Disease: A Profile of Sheffield*. Sheffield: Sheffield Health Authority.

Kamin, Leon (1974). *The Science and Politics of I.Q.* New York: Erlbaum (also Harmondsworth: Penguin, 1977).

Kazdin, Alan (1982). *Single-Case Research Design: Methods for Clinical and Applied Settings*. Oxford: Oxford University Press.

Kelly, George (1955). *The Psychology of Personal Constructs*. New York: Norton.

Kenner, Charmian (1985). *No Time for Women: Exploring Women's Health in the 1930s and Today*. London: Pandora.

Kirkham, Mavis (1983). 'Labouring in the dark: limitations on the giving of information to enable patients to orient themselves to the likely events and timescale of labour', in J. Wilson-Barnett (ed.) *Nursing Research: Ten Studies in Patient Care*. Chichester: Wiley. (A slightly shortened version is reprinted in Abbott and Sapsford, op. cit., 1992.)

Kitzinger, Sheila (1978). *Women as Mothers*. London: Fontana.

Knight, Barry and West, Donald (1975). 'Temporary and continuing delinquency' *British Journal of Criminology*, 15: 43.

Kratz, Charlotte (ed.) (1979). *The Nursing Process*. London: Baillière Tindall.

Lorenson, Margarethe (1983). 'Effects of touch in patients during a crisis situation in hospital', in J. Wilson-Barnett (ed.) *Nursing Research: Ten Studies in Patient Care*. Chichester: Wiley.

McClelland, D., Atkinson, V.W., Clarke, R.A. and Lowell, E.L. (1953). *The Achievement Motive*. New York: Appleton Century.

McCracken, Grant (1988). *The Long Interview*. Beverly Hills: Sage.

McKee, Paul (1981). *Statistics of Politics*, in Open University Course D291 *Statistical Sources*. Milton Keynes: The Open University.

McLeod, C.J. and Slodatski, A.N. (1978). 'How to find out: a guide to searching the nursing literature' *Nursing Times*, 74/6: 21–3.

Marsh, Catherine (1982). *The Survey Method: The Contribution of Surveys to Sociological Explanation*. London: Allen and Unwin.

Marsh, Catherine (1988). *Exploring Data: An Introduction to Data Analysis for Social Scientists*. Cambridge: Polity.

Marsh, G.N. and Channing D.M. (1986). 'Deprivation and health in one General Practice' *British Medical Journal*, 292: 1173–6.

Maternity Services Advisory Committee (1984). *Maternity Care in Action Pt II: Care during Childbirth*. London: HMSO.

Maternity Services Advisory Committee (1985). *Maternity Care in Action Pt III: Care of the Mother and Baby*. London: HMSO.

Metcalf, Clare (1983). 'A study of change in the method of organising the delivery of nursing care in a ward of a maternity hospital', in J. Wilson-Barnett (ed.) op. cit.

Mies, Maria (1983). 'Towards a methodology for feminist research', in G. Bowles and R. Klein (eds) op. cit.

Mitchell, J. Clyde (1983). 'Case and situation analysis' *Sociological Review*, 31: 187–211.
Nairn, Kathy and Smith, Gerrilyn (1984). *Dealing with Depression*. London: Women's Press.
Newmark, Charles (1985). *Major Psychological Assessment Instruments*. Boston: Allyn and Bacon.
Oakley, Ann (1972). *Sex, Gender and Society*. London: Fontana.
Oakley, Ann (1980). *Women Confined: Towards a Sociology of Childbirth*. Oxford: Martin Robertson.
Oakley, Ann (1981). *From Here to Maternity*. Harmondsworth: Penguin.
Office of Population Censuses and Surveys (various). *OPCS Monitor*. London: OPCS.
Office of Population Censuses and Surveys (annual). *Population Trends*. London: HMSO.
Office of Population Censuses and Surveys (annual). *Social Trends*. London: HMSO.
Oja, Sharon and Smulyan, Lisa (1988). *Collaborative Action Research: A Developmental Process*. Basingstoke: Falmer.
Orr, Jean (1986). 'Working with women's health groups: the community health movement', in A. While (ed.) *Research in Preventive Community Nursing: Fifteen Studies in Health Visiting*. Chichester: Wiley. (A shortened version is reprinted in Abbott and Sapsford, op. cit., 1992.)
Jean Orr (ed.) (1987) *Women's Health in the Community*. Chichester: Wiley.
Osgood, Charles, Sui, George and Tannenbaum, Percy (1967). *The Measurement of Meaning*. Urbana (Illinois): University of Illinois Press.
Patton, Michael (1987). *How to Use Qualitative Methods in Evaluation*. Beverly Hills: Sage.
Penfold, Susan and Walker, Gillian (1984). *Women and the Psychiatric Paradox*. Milton Keynes: Open University Press.
Plummer, Kenneth (1983). *Documents of Life: An Introduction to the Problems and Literature of a Humanistic Method*. London: Allen and Unwin.
Polgar, Stephen and Thomas, Shane (1988). *Introduction to Research in the Health Sciences*. London: Churchill Livingstone.
Porter, Marilyn (1983). *Home, Work and Class Consciousness*. Manchester: Manchester University Press.
Pryce, Ken (1979). *Endless Pressure: A Study of West Indian Life-styles in Bristol*. Harmondsworth: Penguin.
Reason, Peter (1981). 'An exploration in the dialectics of two-person relationships', in P. Reason and J. Rowan (eds) op. cit.
Reason, Peter and Rowan, John (eds) (1981). *Human Inquiry: A Sourcebook of New Paradigm Research*. Chichester: Wiley.
Reinharz, Shulamit (1979). *On Becoming a Social Scientist*. San Francisco: Jossey-Bass.
Reinharz, Shulamit (1983). 'Experiential analysis: a contribution to feminist research', in G. Bowles and R. Klein (eds) op. cit.
Roethlisberger, F.J. and Dickson, W.J. (1939). *Management and the Worker*. Harvard: Harvard University Press.
Rose, Nikolas (1985). *The Psychological Complex*. London: Routledge and Kegan Paul.
Rose, Stephen and Black, Bruce (1985). *Advocacy and Empowerment: Mental Health Care in the Community*. London: Routledge and Kegan Paul.
Ross, H.L. and Campbell, D.T. (1968). 'The Connecticut speed crackdown: a study of the effects of legal change', in H.L. Ross (ed.) *Perspectives on the Social Order: Readings in Sociology*. New York: McGraw-Hill.
Roth, Julius (1963). *Timetables*. Indianapolis: Bobbs-Merril.

Sapsford, Roger (1983). *Life-sentence Prisoners: Reaction, Response and Change.* Milton Keynes: Open University Press.

Sapsford, Roger and Thomas, Kerry (1985). 'Change, the individual and the social world' in Block 7 of Open University course D307 *Social Psychology: Development, Experience and Behaviour.* Milton Keynes: The Open University.

Savage, Wendy (1986). *A Savage Enquiry: Who Controls Childbirth?* London: Virago.

Shearer, Anne (1972). *A Report on Public and Professional Attitudes towards the Sexual and Emotional Attitudes of Handicapped People.* London: Spastics Society/National Association for Mental Handicap.

Sherlock, Effie (1987). 'The Liverpool experience: the Croxteth Women's health Group – self-help on a deprived community of Liverpool', in Jean Orr (ed.) op. cit.

Shotter, John (1975). *Images of Man in Psychological Research.* London: Methuen.

Smith, Dorothy (1987). *The Everyday World as Problematic: A Feminist Sociology.* Boston: Northeastern Universities Press.

Tandon, Rajesh (1981). 'Dialogue as enquiry and intervention', in P. Reason and J. Rowan (eds) op. cit.

Taylor, S.J. and Bogden R. (1984). *An Introduction to Qualitative Research Methods: The Search for Meanings.* Chichester: Wiley.

Torbert, William (1981). 'A collaborative enquiry into voluntary metropolitan desegregation', in P. Reason and J. Rowan (eds) op. cit.

Townsend, Peter and Davidsons, N. (eds) (1990). *Inequalities in Health.* Harmondsworth: Penguin.

Townsend, Peter *et al.* (1985). 'Inequalities in health in the city of Bristol: a preliminary review of statistical evidence' *International Journal of Health Science,* 15: 637–63.

Townsend, Peter, Phillimore, P. and Beattie, A. (1986a). *Inequalities in Health in the Northern Region: An Interim Report.* Northern Regional Health Authority.

Townsend, Peter *et al.* (1986b). *Poverty and the London Labour Market: An Interim Report.* London: Low Pay Unit.

Voysey, M. (1975). *A Constant Burden: The Reconstitution of Family Life.* London: Routledge and Kegan Paul.

Wellmer, Albrecht (1969). *Critical Theory of Society.* New York: Herder and Herder.

West, Donald (1967). *Who Becomes Delinquent?* London: Heinemann.

West, Donald (1969). *Present Conduct and Future Delinquency.* London: Heinemann.

West, Donald and Farrington, David (1975). *The Delinquent Way of Life.* London: Heinemann.

Whitehead, M. (1987). *The Health Divide: Inequalities in Health in the 1980s.* London: Health Education Council.

Williams, Anne (1987). 'Making sense of feminist contributions to women's health', in Jean Orr (ed.) op. cit.

Williams, Paul and Shoultz, Bonnie (1982). *We Can Speak for Ourselves: Self-advocacy by Mentally Handicapped People.* London: Souvenir Press.

Wilson-Barnett, Jenifer and Robinson, Sarah (eds) (1989). *Directions in Nursing Research.* Harrow: Scutari.

Witts, L.J. (ed.) (1964). *Medical Surveys and Clinical Trials.* London: Oxford University Press.

Index

abortion statistics, 83
action research, 41, 101–3, 104, 143
advocacy, 146–7
affective flattening, 96
age, 4, 67
analysing qualitative data, 117–26
analytic induction, 129
appraisal, 142
attitude scales, 94–5, 99–100
attitudes, 61, 93–6
autobiography, 133, 134

battered women, see 'domestic' violence
behaviourism, 145
birth statistics, 75, 82
Black Report, 69, 75
blocking, 69

cancer statistics, 83
car ownership, 70, 72
case analysis, 119–20
case control, 53, 62, 106–7
census, 10, 55, 65, 71, 74, 82
centrality, 109
child abuse, 50–2
co-counselling, 142
coding, 12
cohort studies, 60, 88
collaborative research, 98, 110, 134,
    141–7, 161
common sense, limitations of, 3–4,
    161
community care, 27–37
composite measurement, 71
confidentiality, 98

confounded variables, 74, 103
consciousness-raising, 143, 161, 163
content analysis, 120–2
contraception, 159
control, statistical, 66–7, 106
control/comparison groups, 13–14,
    28, 48–9, 53, 56, 136
controlled trial, see experiment
coping strategies, 30, 37
correlation, 68, 73, 74
critical analysis, 124

death statistics, see mortality statistics
defences, 41, 43
depression, 47–50
determinism, 160, 163
diagnosis, 48, 56, 83
disablement statistics, 71
discourse, 161–3
documentary research, 85–6
'domestic' violence, 41, 143
double-blind techniques, 105
drinking, 83

ecological fallacy, 73
ethics
    and confidentiality, 98
    and covert participation, 43,
        129–30
    and experimentation, 15, 104–5,
        146
    and open interviewing, 110
    of research in general, 21–2, 25–6,
        159, 161
    and research on colleagues, 133–4